THE
WOMAN
DOCTOR

THE
WOMAN
DOCTOR

Her Career in Modern Medicine

by Patricia H. Beshiri

COWLES BOOK COMPANY, INC.
NEW YORK

To My Mother and Dr. Jack

PREFACE

The contributions of women to medical manpower needs have been under sharp scrutiny. Surveys have shown that women do as well in medical school as men. They are academically equipped for the training. Surveys have also shown that the dropout rate of women is almost as low as that of men.

Women are good students. Women are good interns and residents, and can contribute to the medical needs of our nation. Women are good doctors. The better and more complete a woman's training after graduation, the easier it is for her to obtain a job compatible with raising a family, or to qualify for any position that might appeal to her if she remains single. By such preparation, the tendency to drop out is automatically reduced. Certain fields, some of them almost unexplored by women, would be most fitting to a married woman's dual career. In spite of this, only 7 percent of the physicians in the United States are women, while 40 percent of the American labor force consists of women.

Plans to mobilize womanpower for the medical professions have been launched by many public and private groups. The result so far has been a statistical answer to a statistical problem. A professional career cannot be handled like a punch card in an organized population survey. A medical career is a deeply personal matter requiring very individualized plans after very critical consideration of many facets far beyond the statistic. Until recently, young women had no place to turn for such personalized information. This book is intended to fill that gap. What are the personal requirements for a medical career as they specifically apply to women? What are the personal experiences of such a career? What are the personal rewards for such effort?

The medical manpower shortage is a "now" problem as well as a future problem of our population's increasing demands. Although there is no instant solution to medical shortages, there is an obvious resource in mobilizing the woman physicians who are not pursuing their careers. Considerable thought and direction have gone into a variety of plans for retraining dropout woman doctors, but the individual candidates have to be reached. The programs must be brought to them, as these women are anchored to their surroundings and cannot seek training just anywhere.

In addition to mobilizing the inactive woman physicians, it is equally urgent that plans be made to reduce the number of women who will be forced into retirement by the inappropriateness of their training or failure to anticipate the problems of combining career and child raising. It is here that we need to take a long look at our present teaching programs and the counseling facilities in our medical schools.

There are those who question the contribution of a woman to medicine, whether in practice, research, or teaching. Especially suspect is the woman with a dual commitment to medicine and marriage. It should be noted that these women have made significant contributions over the years. But far and away more important is that women have made contributions that have not been publicized nor dramatized. One cannot measure the contribution of any physician in hours per day, years per total lifetime, or number of patients seen per unit of time. Is a heart transplant a greater contribution than an immunization given to a child in a clinic? The contributions a woman can make are almost limitless.

The information explosion in all the scientific fields today is tremendous, and in medicine it is beyond comprehension. A medical education is obsolete in five years unless it is constantly revitalized. Every woman doctor must plan for herself a rigorous "keep-in-touch program" that will continue from the moment of graduation, regardless of job or domestic pressure.

Women should not be singled out, nor do they need to band together in a militant crusade. Women in medicine, however, do need to communicate and to share the responsibility of making their contribution to medicine. The medical field cannot afford the luxury of training anyone who will not serve it in some capacity. A woman who accepts a medical degree accepts a personal responsibility to use this knowledge and training. She also accepts a responsibility to the generations of women who will follow her in seeking similar opportunities in the field of medicine.

There is no legislation that forces a woman doctor to use her training. The final responsibility rests with the individual. The surveys, statistics, and reports of individual successes and failures must be followed up with concrete plans and programs that will give every one of them an opportunity to make full use of her training. We must also prepare the women now in college and medical school to plan realistically for the future.

This book is intended to help young women everywhere who are thinking of the medical field as a career to see the role of woman doctors in modern society. It is intended, too, as a source book for guidance counselors and others in a position to help direct someone into a medical career, from high school through to residency. It should lead to more informed preparations and the successful utilization of a great resource—women.

Ruth A. Lawrence, M.D.
Assistant Professor of Pediatrics
The University of Rochester School
of Medicine and Dentistry

ACKNOWLEDGMENTS

It would be an interesting piece of mischief to mention the two or three individuals who failed to cooperate during the extensive research that went into compiling this book. It would certainly be easier than trying to find a suitable way to acknowledge the dozens of people who took hours of time from their busy professional activities. To those who wrote lengthy letters, granted personal interviews, spent time in thoughtful discussions, and followed up with requested material and research, I owe a large debt of thanks.

Dr. Ruth Lawrence has been a continuing source of inspiration throughout the entire project. I thank her not only for the research, papers, and current follow-up studies she provided, but for her guidance, suggestions, and encouragement. Dr. Lawrence kept a steady stream of information pouring into my mailbox throughout the progress of the book, and always had a helpful suggestion when I turned to her for advice. Thanks are also due to other faculty members and students of the University of Rochester (New York) School of Medicine and Dentistry—particularly Dr. James Bartlett—for making me so welcome on their campus and providing pertinent material.

I am very grateful to the University of Miami (Florida) School of Medicine and its facilities. Faced with a constant stream of requests from a resident author, many doctors and staff workers rose to the occasion. After six years as a medical school staff member at Miami, I continued to haunt the labs, libraries, and clinical facilities to gather material for this project. To those who served as interview subjects, answered endless questions, and looked up data, and to the students I met and talked with over the years— thank you.

Without the cooperation and consent of the Association of American Medical Colleges and the studies of Dr. Davis G. Johnson, the American Medical Women's Association and the writings of its *Journal,* and the American Medical Association, particularly Dr. Hayden C. Nicholson, and the material from its *Journal* and other publications, much of the authoritative and factual content of this book would not have been possible.

Mrs. Mary Keyserling, former director of the Women's Bureau of the United States Department of Labor, has been most helpful, as have Dr. Glen R. Leymaster, president of Woman's Medical College of Pennsylvania; Dr. John Z. Bowers, president of the Josiah Macy, Jr., Foundation; and Dr. Margaret L. Brown, curriculum coordinator of the Physician Trainee Program at Pacific Medical Center.

Dr. David Denker, president, and the faculty and staff of New York Medical College also made me most welcome on their campus for repeated visits. Drs. Helen Kaplan and Margaret Giannini offered information, interest, and cooperation.

Thanks are also due to the doctors, educators, and students who granted interviews and presented their stories and opinions candidly, with a sincere desire to help future woman physicians. Many of these people relinquished personal privacy for the sake of the success of these efforts. It is my hope that the reader will benefit from reading about their views, ideas, and programs, and thus the subjects will gain satisfaction from their contributions.

None of the efforts of the many could have been utilized unless the author, as catalyst, could bring such a variety of ideas and opinions to the printed page. During the long months of drafting, writing, and rewriting, my husband Lon has been a steadying force, and Suzy, Lonny, and Gerald have shown patience far beyond their years.

Patricia H. Beshiri

Miami, Florida

CONTENTS

PART I

WOMAN'S ROLE IN THE PRESENT AGE IN MEDICINE

Chapter One

AMERICA'S WASTED RESOURCE

The "glamour" career fields of the space-age physical sciences may be siphoning much of the talent from fields that formerly attracted our nation's top students. "Medicine is not faring well in the midst of this change and development," according to Dr. John M. Stalnaker, president of the National Merit Scholarship Corporation, headquartered in Evanston, Illinois.

"Highly able girls may be a resource which can be used to a greater extent in developing physicians of the future; evidence from other countries supports this possibility," Dr. Stalnaker states in an article published in the *Journal of Medical Education.*[1] When medicine was presented as a career choice to girls of the general population, only 2 percent told NMSC researchers they intended to become physicians.

Although medicine still attracts superior students, and a high IQ is certainly not the only criterion for success, indications are that a "space gap" is developing that will offer greater opportunity to women seeking careers in the still male-dominated medical profession. NMSC studies[2] during the past ten years reflect an "aerospace effect": the nation's top scholars now prefer to pursue Ph.D.'s rather than M.D.'s.

In 1966, for the first time in five years, the number of applicants for admission to the first year of medical school declined.[3] Dr. Stalnaker feels that the problem of obtaining a continuing high level of medical school applicants is increasing, for all except the most prestigious private medical schools.

The United States Public Health Service estimates that the nation will require an additional fifty thousand physicians by 1975.[4] Medical educators bemoan the fact that we are wasting valuable human resources by not encouraging talented women to seek M.D. degrees—yet, when these women do apply, they must face overwhelming odds to be accepted. Only 6 percent of the physicians and surgeons in the United States are women.[5]

It becomes apparent that the United States may practice the harshest discrimination of any country in the world against the woman who wants to become a doctor and still enjoy a balanced life that includes marriage and motherhood. With regard to the increasing number of women entering medical careers throughout the world, America is far below most of the countries of Europe and Asia. With the need for more physicians reaching the critical point, national interest must be focused on attracting qualified women to medicine as a career.

The most dramatic example of the "aerospace effect" in opening up new opportunities for women exists in the Soviet Union. Women dominate the medical profession to such an extent that recent studies show about 75 percent of Russian physicians are female. Dr. John Z. Bowers states, in the *New England Journal of Medicine*,[6] that these figures reflect not only national policy but also personal preference. Since the advent of the space age, medicine has lost the high status it formerly had in the USSR, and the best male students are entering other fields of science, technology, commerce, and industry.

Female enrollments in medical schools throughout western Europe reflect the value these countries place on the contributions of their women to medicine. In France, 27 percent of all medical students and 26 percent of all dental students are women; in Great Britain, 25 percent. Germany has 30 percent female medical school graduates, and the Netherlands 20 percent.

Even the nations we consider "underdeveloped" in Asia and Latin America far surpass the United States in educating their talented young women as doctors. India has 35 percent, Indonesia 30 percent, Korea 25 percent, Brazil 13 percent, and Chile 20 percent. In the United States, 9.1 percent of all medical students are women.[7]

Defenders of the status quo attempt to refute such comparative statistics by criticizing the quality of the medical education in other countries. While many countries admittedly do not equal America in their educational standards and facilities, the important point is that the best they have is being shared by woman students to a greater extent than in the United States. And as the foreign academic systems are being upgraded and extended, the valuable health services of woman doctors are not being lost in the meantime.

It is to be hoped that publication of such studies as the above will make the American people aware that women are needed in medicine. If a country such as India, where women achieved equal opportunity in society only after the end of World War II, can produce a percentage of woman physicians three times greater than the United States, can a more important role in medicine for our emancipated women be far behind?

E. W. Nugent, assistant executive director of the Dade County Medical Association (Greater Miami, Florida), agrees that many men are now being drawn from medicine toward the physical sciences, particularly in aerospace-oriented areas such as Florida.

"The attraction is there, although the other fields are not consciously wooing the students. There is the glamour of the approach to space sciences with all the attendant publicity," Nugent says. "The tremendous expansion of knowledge in the physical sciences is another attraction, particularly to a highly creative and curious intellect."

A recent study published in the *Journal of the American Medical Association*[8] backs this up. The percentage of "A" students in medical schools has declined slightly for the past twelve years, but it has been accompanied by a reduction in the proportion of "C" students. This may reflect two trends: the pull of the new fields on the top scholars, and the growing tendency of medical school admissions committees to consider qualities other than grades in selecting their entering freshmen. (More recently, there has appeared to be increasing dissatisfaction with a description of the "good" medical student based entirely on his grades in medical school. Admissions committees are now directing more attention to students who are personable and emotionally stable and have a broad educational background. These factors are being sought, as well as— or, in some cases, instead of—excellence in scholarship.)

The length of time required to complete a medical education is a deterrent to many considering the profession. If one intends to specialize, he can complete ten years of training after graduating from college and still be just at the threshold of his career. This time factor discourages many men who wish to begin their careers sooner and can do so with a Ph.D.

"To achieve the same level in medicine as in the physical sciences takes much longer," Nugent stated. "The 'union ticket' in the physical sciences is the Ph.D., and this can be acquired in about four years after receiving the bachelor's degree. Most universities grant a stipend to the Ph.D. candidate; so he is already enjoying the satisfaction of teaching and research while completing graduate study." This can be the decisive factor to the married male student, especially if he already has children.

Unlike her male counterpart, a woman does not have to assume the financial burden of supporting her family should she decide to marry during her student years. She can reject the teaching or research fellowship that a man might eagerly accept to give him financial stability. Being free of dependents, she can choose to assume greater loan obligations, which she can pay off in installments when she begins her professional career.

So, while there is no dearth of medical school applicants, women will have an increasing opportunity for acceptance as these trends continue, and the girl with a well-rounded background plus a fistful of "A's" will stand a better chance with admissions committees.

The immediate problem is to garner the talents of the young women qualified for medicine before the potential contribution of their generation is lost. This requires careful career planning and selection of the field in which to practice; a sound educational background; and a healthy emotional attitude toward the special problems women face when they embark on the nine-year program leading to a physician's practice.

Dr. Bowers has consulted with faculty members and administrators concerned with female students in the liberal arts colleges, the premedical phase of education where a girl's interest in a scientific career first crystallizes, in an effort to determine why those who express no interest in medicine have given little serious consideration to it as a career. He has found that many potential female medical students come to believe during their undergraduate years that, in the United States, medicine is not for women.

Female students lose interest in medicine for a number of reasons: a desire for early marriage and a family; the belief that medical education is too long and difficult; the impression that women are not wanted in medical schools; the inflexibility of medical education, especially during internship and residency, with the result that it is almost impossible both to complete the program and have a family; and fear of encountering an antifeminine attitude in the medical establishment.[7]

Women do not realize the diversity available in medicine. They must be informed that an active career in medicine, marriage, and a lively family life are compatible. To go into medicine is not to commit oneself to a single track. In practice, a woman doctor can control her work intake, even in a specialty as demanding as obstetrics. For instance, she can establish a partnership practice with another doctor, man or woman. Girls should realize from the outset that they can limit their practice to a scope that is manageable for a wife and mother.

High school and undergraduate college counselors often influence the career choices of young women. Counselors cannot emphasize too strongly that the earlier a girl decides to enter medicine, the better will be her preparation and the greater her chances for acceptance to medical school. On the other hand, counselors may not be disposed toward medicine; some offer little encouragement or information. A girl should realize, however, that there are other sources of guidance. The local medical association, the family physician, or a sympathetic faculty member of a nearby medical school are among those able to advise a girl who wishes to develop her talent in medical science but is unsure of how to go about it.

Women must learn to approach medicine as a businesslike career, not a state of sainthood. Too many students resign control over their own education, taking only the prescribed courses instead of developing their individual potential. A girl who hopes to enter medicine should investigate during the undergraduate years the possibility of substituting courses that interest her, and should fit them into her premed program. In this way, she can acquire a sound scientific background to apply to a specialty such as pathology, psychiatry, or some other field that she may want to pursue in medicine. Many of these careers have the advantage of regular workaday hours.

Greater participation by all members of the health professions is needed to tackle the problem from every side. The public must be educated to the urgent need for expansion of teaching facilities to train the doctors necessary to serve our population. Women must be motivated to make their special contribution to the profession.

A professor at a large southern medical school (who obviously needs the protection of his requested anonymity) outspokenly reinforces this opinion:

"I think women make better doctors than men. Who makes a good doctor? Someone who is cautious, emotionally interested in people, cares about people, has sympathy. Women seem to have these characteristics as part of their personality makeup. The 'tricky diagnosis'—the intellectual part of medicine which appeals to men—comes up only about once a year. Men are mainly interested in furthering their own careers. Women have the more selfless approach, and this is of great benefit to their patients."

Notes to Chapter One

1. John M. Stalnaker, LL.D., "The Attitudes of High School Students Toward Higher Education," *Journal of Medical Education*, Vol. 38.
2. The Merit Program: The First Decade, 1955:1965, National Merit Scholarship Corporation.
3. *Journal of the American Medical Association*, Vol. 198, No. 8, November 21, 1966. Figures and comparisons also made from same study published in 1965: Davis G. Johnson, Ph.D., "The Study of Applicants, 1964–1965," *Journal of Medical Education*, Vol. 40, November, 1965.
4. *The Opportunities and Rewards of Medicine Can be Yours*, American Medical Association, 1965.
5. *Women in Scientific Careers*, National Science Foundation, 1961.
6. John Z. Bowers, M.D., "Women in Medicine: An International Study," *New England Journal of Medicine*, 275: 362–365, August 18, 1966.
7. *Ibid.*
8. *Ibid.*

Chapter Two

THE PARADOX

The space age, by attracting many of the nation's top male scholars, makes a woman's chances of acceptance to medical school better than ever. Women have already proved that their contributions to the profession can be major ones. As medical students, they are generally accepted by their male peers. The nationwide shortage of physicians is becoming acute.

Why, then, aren't medical educators actively wooing bright young women into the profession? Why is our percentage of female physicians so much lower than that of most other countries? Why do some medical educators openly admit they are against women in medicine?

Shortage of Educational Facilities

Dr. James W. Bartlett, associate dean of the University of Rochester (New York) School of Medicine and Dentistry, defines one of the most critical problems facing our country in this generation:

"I am not for encouraging more women to become medical students. Our country does not have sufficient educational facilities to meet the needs of the qualified students, male or female, who are applying to study medicine today. If a woman cannot participate in medicine full-time for life, she is taking the seat in medical school of a man who *will* do so."

The University of Rochester's medical school is in the fortunate position of being one of the "prestigious private medical schools" to which Dr. Stalnaker referred in Chapter 1. Founded in 1920, richly endowed, and highly regarded in the academic world, it accepts seventy-five freshman medical students each year from more than twelve hundred applicants. About one thousand of these are qualified students, according to Dr. Bartlett.

Support for new educational facilities is needed from many sources: the general public, private endowments, increased government funds, legislation favoring medical education. Enormous quantities of money are available for graduate study in the "space-race professions"—a large part of it, funds that were formerly channeled into medicine and medical research. Meanwhile, here on earth, we are facing a critical shortage of physicians and up-to-date physical plants. Our teaching hospitals must be modernized and faculties increased. Efficiency innovations, such as closed-circuit TV, central records systems, and new equipment, can help us utilize better the personnel we have.

Within the limits of the small classes that now exist, women who apply for admission into medical school are being accepted in nearly the same proportion as men. A recent study published by the *Journal of the American Medical Association*[1] revealed that of women who applied to United States medical schools, 47.7 percent were accepted for admission. This compares with an acceptance rate of 48.2 percent of male applicants. It is just that far too few are applying—and there is precious little space for those who do.

Doctor Dropouts

Dr. Davis G. Johnson, director of student affairs of the Association of American Medical Colleges, speaks out for the educators who think that women may already be taking enough seats in medical schools:

"Studies by our Association indicate that women do not *practice* medicine to anywhere near the extent of men." [2]

Dr. Johnson does not see much increased opportunity for women in medicine until their attrition rate can be reduced. Such attrition includes the gradual wearing down of a woman's resources and motivation that finally leads her to opt for marriage instead of—not in conjunction with—medicine.

Most of the dropping out seems to occur after medical school has been completed, and this is the most pointed argument of those who question women's desire to be part of the medical profession. E. W. Nugent, who thinks the space age will open wider the medical field for women, expresses this concern about a female doctor's contribution in the early years of her career:

"There is a steadily increasing number of women in the classes of most medical schools. More women want to go into medicine now than in the past. The only trouble is—most do not stay in the field for any length of time. They finish the education, then get married, have a family, and either practice part-time or drop out of the profession until their families are grown. There is this hiatus . . . when the children are young."

With knowledge in medical science expanding so rapidly, it is difficult for a practicing physician, research worker, or professor to keep abreast of new developments. For a doctor-wife and mother who abandons medicine even temporarily, it is still more difficult.

A study made by the Association of American Medical Colleges[3] found that a higher percentage of men (92 percent) than women (84 percent) completed their medical education. Most of the men who dropped out, however, did so because of academic problems. More than half of the women who dropped out did so for other reasons, including marriage and pregnancy.

"The woman medical student becomes a public resource; society has a tremendous investment in her," Dr. Bartlett states emphatically.

She is already in debt to society when she takes her seat as a freshman medical student. Does this mean, then, that marriage, children, or even dating must be sacrificed to the rarefied air of academe as the medical school coed turns into a grind?

Cathy Tullsen thinks the social life in medical school is great! A pretty brown-haired sophomore at the University of Rochester School of Medicine, she admits to having more dates now than in her undergraduate years. Yet—and she is on scholarship—her grades are not suffering.

"You can manage both dating and studies. I prefer to date medical students because they understand when I have to refuse an invitation in order to study. But we arrange our social life around the demands of the academic load and manage to have plenty of fun."

Cathy intends to specialize and wants to combine marriage with her career. "I do not think it is fair to drop completely out of practice during the child-raising years. You can never leave the profession, even for a short time."

Cathy realizes how quickly knowledge can become outdated in this fast-moving scientific age. She feels she can always keep her hand in, working part-time while the children are young and staying abreast of the literature and new developments in her field.

"In choosing a specialty, I will try to select one with regular hours. For me, this would automatically exclude obstetrics." She considers pathology one field that is both fascinating and ideal for a family woman.

Cathy Tullsen is the kind of girl Dr. Bartlett encourages to enter medical school. She admits that she is not as idealistic as she was in college: "A lot of my missionary zeal has abated." Cathy realizes medicine is a job, not the road to canonization. But she thinks being able to work for a lifetime in a profession that has absorbed her for years will compensate for the long hours of study and hard work now.

"I feel very responsible for being accepted to medical school" is the way Cathy explains her determination to succeed. "I am taking the place of a man who would have worked just as hard and practiced full-time. I never forget this."

The Mother-Doctor's Contribution

The total contribution a woman doctor makes throughout her life was examined at a recent conference on "The Fuller Utilization of the Woman Physician." It was found that, although many women drop out of medicine, at least part-time, to have children, they remain out of active practice a relatively short period if contact with the profession is maintained. Attention is now being given to the lifetime working pattern of woman doctors, who have many productive years ahead once their children are through elementary school. Those whose families are raised can readily return to their work full-time if they have kept current, or if they can take a retraining program to update their skills.

This is true of women throughout the labor force in today's society. "Over 50% of all women aged 45 to 55 are now employed . . . more than half of all women 45 to 55 years old are now actively in the labor force. In other words, it is the older women, not the younger ones, who are most likely to be working—an amazing fact, which exposes so many old entrenched ideas . . . the years past the age of 40 were unquestionably assumed to be high-risk years fraught with danger and instability. Today there is great regard for the middle-aged female worker." [4]

Medical education is not, therefore, being wasted on a woman who wishes to fulfill her feminine role as wife and mother. In fact, the more education she has in any field, the more likely she is to work. Dr. Eli Ginzberg pointed out at the conference that "the more education they have, the shorter the period they stay out of the labor force. This seems to be a persistent trend: more and more women wish to remain at work even while they have young children at home, and this tendency is reinforced with increased educational level." [5]

In medicine, group practice, salaried positions, and less-than-full-time jobs employ disproportionate numbers of women today. Extension of these opportunities will attract even more women and keep them active in the profession.

And the time spent at home raising children is not a professional loss to the mother-doctor. Dr. Dorothy V. Whipple, a pediatrician, points out the value of motherhood as an integral part of medical training:

"A few years spent at home by the highly trained professional doctor need not be considered wasted years. . . . Not only do the children have a mother's care, but the doctor herself learns things she can never learn in any school. She comes to know, because she has experienced, the pleasure of watching a child balance the top block on his tower . . . she knows the boredom and loneliness of home chores and home confinement; maybe she experiences the soul-chilling fear of watching beside a seriously ill child.

"This knowledge is of infinite value to any doctor who ultimately deals with people. It provides the basis of an empathy which is an essential ingredient in the art of medicine. The practice of medicine is not all a matter of biochemistry. A few years at home . . . bring rich rewards in understanding. It is only women who are given the opportunity for this kind of learning." [6]

More information is needed about the identifiable professional working hours of women doctors and whether, in addition, some may be volunteering uncounted hours of professional service in committee work and other contributions to the community well-being.[7] The brief child-raising hiatus may be comparable to the military obligations of male physicians, and perhaps the problem of the child-bearing doctor dropout has been overemphasized in comparing the lifetime working patterns of male and female physicians.

Once a doctor, "you can't quit." This is the consensus of educators, practitioners, research workers, and students. Even a temporary hiatus is disastrous to a woman's medical career *if the loss of contact with her profession is complete*. While the children are young, a medical mother can lighten her load considerably and even withdraw from active practice without squandering her hard-won education.

"This little time-out does not mean she makes less of a total contribution than a man," says one professor in defense of mother-doctors. "You do have a career obligation in medicine, because of the limited amount of people who can be educated right now. But a woman can make her own special contribution to the profession. Women have a different makeup and can adjust to the little annoyances. Mothers learn at home to put up with a constant stream of minor aggravations—this trains them to do some of the jobs that do not interest men."

But the paradox persists. Women are needed in medicine. The space age offers them increasing opportunities in the profession. Women belong in medicine, for they have a contribution to make that is unique and should be exploited, rather than trying to cram them into an educational mold designed "for men only." Our nation needs far more physicians than existing medical schools can provide. Yet there is resistance to recruiting the young women whose skills are so urgently needed.

New goals for educators must now be set. Women must not be content to wait for their talents to be utilized at some utopian date when there will be more facilities than male students can use. The solution lies somewhere between the two views shown here. Right now, the limitations are of faculty and space, not of prospective students. Even as these limitations are eased, it is expected that the attraction of other careers, such as the space-age physical sciences, may cause shortages of qualified medical students. At that time, the growing interest of women in careers in medicine will be of critical national importance. Or we can begin now to train our potential woman doctors, and avoid the crisis.

Notes to Chapter Two

1. *Journal of the American Medical Association,* Vol. 198, No. 8, November 21, 1966. Figures and comparisons also made from same study published in 1965: Davis G. Johnson, Ph.D., "The Study of Applicants, 1964 to 1965," *Journal of Medical Education,* Vol. 40, November, 1965.
2. Letter from Davis G. Johnson, December 30, 1966.
3. Datagram on "Women in Medical School," Association of American Medical Colleges, February, 1966.
4. Eli Ginzberg, Ph.D., "Professional Manpower for an Affluent Society: The Opportunity Gap," from report of conference on Meeting Medical Manpower Needs: The Fuller Utilization of the Woman Physician,

January 12–13, 1968, Washington, D.C. Sponsored by American Medical Women's Association, the President's Study Group on Careers for Women, Women's Bureau of U.S. Department of Labor. Report published by American Medical Women's Association, 1968. Pp. 3–7. Reprinted by permission.
5. *Ibid.*
6. Dorothy V. Whipple, M.D., "Practice and Family Life," *op. cit.* Pp. 33–34.
7. "Recommendations," *op. cit.* P. 91.

Chapter Three

PREPARING FOR A CAREER IN MEDICINE

One of the most frequently voiced regrets of women in medicine —and women who wish they were—is, "If only I had started sooner."

Woman students and physicians are unanimous in emphasizing the importance of making the career decision early in one's education, in order to dispel the aura of mystery and holiness of purpose that surrounds the word "doctor" and discourages many intelligent, qualified women from considering the field.

Can You Take Medicine?

If you are a young woman who aspires to the medical profession, ask yourself the following questions. The answers will help you evaluate your potential as a doctor. In the event that you can't come up with satisfactory answers for some of them, keep in mind that it takes years to develop the desirable qualities discussed below, and that they represent the ideal in a physician's personality. If you are still several years away from entering medical school, there is plenty of time to mature and train yourself for greater responsibilities. If you are ready to embark on your career and find yourself seriously deficient in these desirable traits, the knowledge may direct you to the most suitable branch of medicine, or away from the profession entirely. There are alternatives to a physician's practice, such as research or teaching, that permit participation in medical careers by a wide variety of personalities.

1. Are you a good student? Because of continual advances in science and medicine, a doctor's education never ends. In addition to the time spent in school to obtain an M.D. (or Ph.D.), a doctor must be prepared for a lifetime of reading texts, publications, and papers. Above-average intelligence is required to assimilate, retain, and apply the complex scientific material.

This does not mean you cannot make it without having "A" grades. The American Medical Association states[1] that scholastic achievement is only one way of measuring a student's capacity for success in the study of medicine, and that the majority (75 percent) of freshman medical students in the past five years were "B" students. However, in light of the competition for positions in entering classes, the "A" can be quite persuasive.

2. Can you organize your studies and follow through on assignments? If you are a girl who is always in a flap when a term paper is due, who puts off assignments or loses her notes, you will have to do some serious shoring up before attempting a medical career. Rigid self-discipline is necessary in medical school to keep abreast of the course work. A daily study routine must be worked out, and the student must stick with it throughout the academic year. Developing this discipline in high school will result in good study habits, higher grades, and the possibility of accelerating at the lower levels, if you are an above-average student. It is not the difficulty of the curriculum that makes medical school so demanding, but the sheer volume of material to be absorbed, comprehended, and memorized. Without organization and concentration, the student will quickly fall behind.

3. Do you have good health? Good health, both physical and mental, is a must for a doctor. It will enable you to stand up to the strain of long years of study, sometimes combined with part-time work. It will help you to maintain a high interest in your studies and to give full attention to your training. When one feels tired or ill, it is difficult to overlook aggravations, to concentrate on studies, and to maintain the patience required in dealing with people. A physician's practice makes demands on physical health and emotional self-control that are not found in any other profession.

4. Do you like people? It would take a biblical incantation to elaborate all the qualities a physician is required to exhibit when dealing with patients: compassion, tolerance, patience, humanitarianism, warmth, understanding, dedication . . . the list is endless. And these qualities must be combined with the ability to avoid an emotional approach to medicine. Sufficient objectivity must be maintained so that you do not become too involved with your patient's problems to treat him properly.

By their very makeup, women seem to have an advantage in bringing warmth and understanding to the doctor-patient relationship. It is important for a doctor to have compassion and an interest in helping others, never letting people become a series of medical statistics. Each patient is different; he displays his unique symptoms and responds to treatment in his own way. A sincere interest in people as individuals is as much a part of medicine as scientific knowledge is.

5. *Are you realistic?* As one intern put it after her first few hectic weeks on the wards: "If you go into medicine expecting undying gratitude from your patients, forget it. If you think you are going to discover a great cure, forget it. There is more than one way to be dedicated, and I think the hard-work, not the emotional, approach is the right one."

Premedical Preparation in High School

The American Medical Association recommends the following basic courses to be taken for high school credit[2] (they are required by most colleges for any student wishing to enter a liberal arts course, whether in preparation for medicine or another career):

> Four years of English
> Two to three years of laboratory science: chemistry, biology, physics
> Two to four years of modern foreign or classical language
> Three years of mathematics: two of algebra, one of plane geometry
> Two to three years of social studies: history, sociology, economics, political science

Students are urged to enlarge upon these basic requirements by choosing elective courses that will broaden their background in the communication arts. Subjects of individual interest, such as psychology, literature, history, religion, and creative writing, should be explored to develop intellectual abilities. Study to get depth from your course material; it is not enough to skim over subjects just to get by.

Development of your personality, your ability to work with others, and your enjoyment of all types of people is equally important. Participate in extracurricular activities, service organizations, or clubs that interest you. Attend career-day programs when they are offered by your local medical association or community health organization. Volunteer work, after-school or summer jobs, and special study programs are all valuable in learning to accept responsibility.

Participation in your school's science club and its annual science fair is especially valuable to your premedical preparation. The projects of these clubs will stimulate your interest in scientific and medical research and show you the many opportunities for creativity and innovation available in medicine. Further information can be obtained by writing to:

Science Service
1719 N Street, N.W.
Washington, D.C. 20036

Many local medical associations sponsor future physicians' clubs, or paramedical clubs. In cooperation with school officials, these clubs offer an opportunity for the student interested in a medical career to learn about the profession through lectures by physicians in different fields, tours of medical facilities, and observation of doctors at work. Students may accompany a doctor on his rounds, watch surgery being performed, visit a laboratory or a hospital emergency room, and become acquainted with a variety of medical procedures. In addition, guidance is given in the form of information on scholarships, careers allied to medicine, part-time jobs in the health field, and preparation for medical school.

The future doctors' clubs, organized by Kiwanis clubs, and the Ars Medica clubs, sponsored by the American Academy of General Practice, are similar to those sponsored by medical associations. All seek to encourage qualified students to examine the advantages of a medical career and familiarize themselves with the profession. To be eligible for membership, a student must maintain at least a "B" average in his high school studies and be interested in the biological sciences.

The American Academy of General Practice distributes a bimonthly publication, *Ars Medica,* to students participating in its more than fifty clubs. You may obtain copies of current issues by writing to the academy at:

> Volker Boulevard at Brookside
> Kansas City, Missouri 64112

Acceleration—Pro and Con

The official academic view and that of the personal-experience school are far apart in the matter of lower level (premedical school) acceleration of studies. Most educators believe that maturity is gained gradually, from both experience and as wide a base of liberal education as possible. Most medical schools recommend that a student complete the full four years of undergraduate training, and many states will not permit even the most gifted student to accelerate at the high school level.

The premedical sudent must complete at least three full years of undergraduate study (ninety credits) to meet the minimum academic requirements of most of the country's medical schools. Four years of college, with or without a bachelor's degree, are considered a plus factor when evaluating a medical school applicant. Thirteen medical schools in the United States require their applicants to have four years of undergraduate study, with or without the degree. The requirements of specific schools are given in Chapter 7.

Despite the objections of educators, the majority of women who are already in the profession, or who have coped with the dual role of wife and mother plus that of medical student, recommend acceleration. These women speak from personal experience and use the common-sense argument that it is easier to shorten your studies by more diligent application in high school and college than it is after you are married, when you are trying to study and run a home at the same time. This approach should be considered seriously by every girl who makes the commitment to a career in medicine.

Acceleration at the high school level is possible in some states for the above-average student. If a girl is mature and responsible in her study habits, she can gain a year in high school and start her nine years of medical study one year sooner.

High school students can take college courses during the summer. The student attends an accredited college (not necessarily the one he will attend after graduation) and takes college-level courses, for college credit, prior to high school graduation. If you have already selected your premedical college, you have an advantage in that you can plan your summer program with your college adviser and be certain of transferring your credits after you graduate from high school. The extra credits will give you the opportunity to take a wider variety of college courses than you normally would have time for, and to explore fields of particular interest that may not fit conveniently into a structured degree program.

You can accelerate at the college level by attending school the year round, including summer sessions. With such a college program it is possible to complete the minimum ninety credits, or even earn a degree, in three years if you always carry the maximum number of credits permitted. Colleges on the trimester system have such a program in effect.

In deciding for or against acceleration, your long-range goal should be the determinant. If there is no particular urgency in completing your education, the traditional program could be the best one for you. If the money available for your education is limited, a year less in college will ease the financial burden. If you are planning to combine marriage and the practice of medicine, it will be far easier to buckle down to a heavy study load before taking on the responsibility of a family. All accelerated programs are open only to the above-average student.

Premedical Preparation in College

You can exercise wide latitude in choosing a premedical college. The college or university you decide upon should be accredited by one of the regional agencies of the American Council on Education. Although this is not mandatory in order for you to receive consideration by a medical school, it is recommended so that you can avoid difficulties in the evaluation of your undergraduate premed credits.

Most high school and college counselors, as well as school and public libraries, have copies of a publication entitled *Universities and Colleges in the United States* available for your reference. This book, which lists all the accredited schools in the United States, may also be obtained by writing to:

American Council on Education
1785 Massachusetts Avenue, N.W.
Washington, D.C. 20036

The national and regional accrediting agencies are:

National Committee of Regional Accrediting Agencies
Middle States Association of Colleges and Secondary Schools
New England Association of Colleges and Secondary Schools
North Central Association of Colleges and Secondary Schools
Northwest Association of Secondary and Higher Schools
Southern Association of Colleges and Secondary Schools
Western College Association

You should select a college of arts and sciences that offers all the required courses you will need to enter medical school. The quality of the science faculty and of the laboratory facilities is of primary importance. Talk to counselors, your family physician, and science teachers to determine if the college you are considering has a high reputation for its academic standards, science departments, and faculty.

Do not plan to utilize junior college credits for your premedical requirements in the sciences. It is advisable to plan on attending only a senior college of arts and sciences. However, if finances or other important considerations make it imperative for you to attend a junior college for part of your undergraduate studies, arrange your schedule so that the major portion of the required sciences will be carried at the senior college level. Many junior colleges have weak science departments; their courses often are composed of survey material that skims over two or three of the basic sciences in one semester, and this is not acceptable to medical school admissions committees. No more than sixty hours of junior college work are accepted by medical schools, and an application that presents only a junior college academic record will not be considered.

Pick a college that fits your personality and social needs, and offers a rich variety of courses for a broad liberal arts background. There are many excellent small colleges of arts and sciences that give students more personalized attention than the multiversities. Some students prefer the stimulation of a large university and the opportunity it affords to meet many different types of students. Being on a university campus that has a medical school is another attraction to consider.

You may find that your state university will be less costly, or perhaps a local school that permits you to live at home and cut down on the expenses of room and board may be desirable. All these factors should be carefully evaluated along with the type of education you desire.

During your last two years of high school, write to several colleges that appeal to you and request their announcement bulletins. Consult the following publications, available in public and school libraries, for accurate and comparative listings:

American Universities and Colleges (10th edition), published by the American Council on Education

Comparative Guide to American Colleges 1968–69, by Cass and Birnbaum, published by Harper & Row

The College Blue Book, by Christian Burckel, published by The College Blue Book, Yonkers, New York

The New American Guide to Colleges, by Gene Hawes, published by Columbia University Press, New York City

These publications will familiarize you with many schools that are not only academically satisfactory but often do not have the plethora of applicants that the larger and better-known colleges attract. Inquire whether the college has a premedical advisory program. If possible, visit some of the colleges you are considering.

The ACAC College Admissions Center. The Association of College Admissions Counselors has established the College Admissions Center as a clearinghouse designed to make the admissions process easier for the student, his counselor, and the college. It requires one registration and one low at-cost fee.

The center employs a sophisticated computerized procedure that matches the student's individual needs and credentials with the admissions criteria of member colleges of the Association of College Admissions Counselors (ACAC).

The center presents the names of new student registrants to the colleges every two weeks. It serves any student seeking undergraduate admission to college, as a freshman or a transfer, matching a student registrant's credentials to the colleges and universities for which he is qualified. The colleges then write directly to the student.

If you wish to use this service, write to the center for a registration form, and complete it in the same way as you would a college application. Return the completed form, along with your academic records from secondary school and college and the nonrefundable fee of twenty dollars. The credentials are reviewed by admissions officers from colleges and universities that use the center's services.

Schools using the center include large state universities, independent universities, small independent colleges, junior colleges, and specialized institutes. All these colleges are fully accredited, except for a few selected new ones that are in the process of achieving accreditation and qualifying according to the stipulations of ACAC's executive board. Premedical students must be sure to notify the center at the time they register that they plan to enter medical school and will require an accredited school with a suitable premedical program.

Although the center does no counseling, ACAC member colleges throughout the United States will provide admissions counseling for returning armed forces veterans, Peace Corps workers, and Vista volunteers who request it. Special rosters have been prepared for Upward Bound students and for an Educational Guidance and Opportunities group of indigent students.

The center does not directly help students to get financial aid, but a student should indicate his financial need on the center's registration form. The individual college admissions officer and his school's financial aid committee will then determine if financial help can be granted.

Although a student may apply to the center at any time within the school year prior to his entrance into college, application by December 1 is desirable. The center's first mailing of potential fall registrants to the colleges is early in November, and new student listings are sent out every two weeks thereafter through the following August. Since January, 1969, high school juniors planning ahead toward college have been permitted to utilize the ACAC-CAC to explore the many realistic admission possibilities. Each participating college receives a separate bimonthly roster of junior registrants who show promise of meeting the college's criteria for admissions, and the school then communicates directly with the students.

As of October, 1969, service for graduate students is being initiated by ACAC-CAC.

For more information write to:

ACAC College Admissions Center
801 Davis Street
Evanston, Illinois 60201

Other organizations that will help students find enrollment are:

College Admissions Assistance Center
41 East 65th Street
New York, New York 10021

Private College Admissions Center (formerly Catholic College Admissions and Information Center)
3805 McKinley Street, N.W.
Washington, D.C. 20015

When you have compared academic programs, tuition costs, living costs in different locations (i.e., in a big city, in a small college town, or on a residential campus), and the quality of the faculty, there is one more important factor to consider. The American Medical Association recommends that you find out the answer to the following question:

"Regardless of size, does the college consistently send some students on to medical school? As a rule, students from colleges that provide several medical students per year are more successful in medical school than students from colleges that contribute only an occasional medical student." [3]

Premedical College Curriculum. The American Medical Association states that most medical schools expect their applicants to have completed courses in biology, physics, inorganic and organic chemistry, the humanities, and the social sciences. Courses in mathematics are recommended for their value in increasing the student's understanding of the laboratory sciences. Medical school applicants should also study English, in order to increase their ability to read comprehensively and to communicate and express their ideas well.

Some colleges offer special premedical programs. Students also may choose to major in such fields as biology or the physical sciences. Medical schools keep their premed requirements to a minimum in order to give the student the best possible opportunity to explore a wide range of subject material and gain a broad background in the arts and sciences.

By the time you are ready to enter your junior year in college, you should know the specific entrance requirements of the medical schools you are considering. Once you have made the decision to enter the medical profession, you should obtain a copy of *Medical School Admission Requirements* from:

Association of American Medical Colleges
2530 Ridge Avenue
Evanston, Illinois 60201

(This publication costs four dollars per copy, postpaid.) Reference copies are available in the offices of guidance counselors and faculty advisers, and in school and public libraries.

Another publication available in the offices of most high school and college guidance counselors is *Horizons Unlimited,* published by the American Medical Association. The book is designed primarily for high school students and beginning college students, and it covers the field of medicine and allied careers. If you are not able to secure a copy locally, write directly to: American Medical Association, 535 North Dearborn Street, Chicago, Illinois 60610.

Notes to Chapter Three

1. *Horizons Unlimited,* American Medical Association, 1968. Pp. 14, 25.
2. *Ibid.*
3. *Op. cit.* P. 20.

Chapter Four

MEDICINE AND MOTHERHOOD

Managing a medical career and a home requires the ability to get organized and stay organized without becoming bogged down in detail. A woman must decide what is most important to each role, and then use her time and energy to accomplish these essentials.

"Women have a different makeup and can do some of the jobs that are not of interest to men, because they learn at home to adjust to the little annoyances.

"I once read an article by a writer who advised career women with children not to let themselves get upset by the minor crises that inevitably arise each day when you are trying to work, take care of children, and manage a home at the same time. As she put it, 'Don't sweat the small stuff.' Conserve your energy for real emergencies and big problems. You can manage a family and a career in medicine if you remember not to 'sweat the small stuff!' "

Quoted is Dr. Ruth Lawrence, who knows whereof she speaks. She is the mother of nine children, ranging from teen age to infancy. She and her husband are both full-time faculty members at the University of Rochester School of Medicine.

Dr. Lawrence married after completing her internship and had her pediatric residency interrupted by the arrival of her first baby. Babies have been interrupting schedules in the Lawrence family ever since. Both of the Drs. Lawrence—he is associate professor of anesthesia—concentrate on teaching careers that allow for hours compatible with family life.

"I am away from home only four or five hours a day. I do here on campus only what cannot be done away, such as teaching and attending to hospital duties. I read, open my mail, and accomplish everything else possible in my home. This eliminates such things as coffee breaks, but it also gets me home by the time school is out for my five oldest children. You must accept and plan around the restrictions imposed by your own environment if you want the privilege of a family."

Dr. Lawrence thinks that the length of a medical education frightens most girls. To her, the most urgent need is getting to young women the information they need on the best way to plan for their careers. They must know what work is available in the field of medicine that will coincide with a happy family life.

"Women can limit their participation while the children are young. As the children grow up, they can contribute more. This brief compromise should not deter a woman from choosing medicine. It is what she brings to the total experience that makes her training valuable."

Ruth Lawrence specializes in care of the newborn. She is in charge of the nursery at Highland Hospital, Rochester, New York. She lectures and teaches her specialty on the wards to students in their clinical years. Although qualified to have a private practice in pediatrics, she currently limits herself to seeing patients only on consultation at local hospitals, and those referred to her by other physicians.

"What with my nine children and those of my friends, I have a large enough sideline practice, although not a very profitable one," she laughs.

Dr. Lawrence participated in the Josiah Macy Foundation conference on "Women for Medicine." The nationally prominent delegates, men and women in education, medicine, and the arts and sciences, considered such pertinent social questions as: Should we have more women in medicine? Are we educating enough women to medicine? Are girls being discouraged from entering medicine during their undergraduate years?

At the Macy conference, Dr. Lawrence spoke on the internship and residency training of women, who are likely to enter these demanding years coincident with marriage and the arrival of the first child. She presented a paper that stressed the special problems of a woman with a young family during these important training years. "I explored programs now being piloted in this area and highlighted my paper with references to my own experience," she recalls.

In preparing her paper, Dr. Lawrence conducted a survey of the woman graduates of the University of Rochester School of Medicine, matching her data wherever possible with that of a previous survey by the university's Medical Education Committee to obtain a significant sample. Her findings included information on the marital status, number of children, amount of postgraduate training, and specialty of the women surveyed. She particularly sought material regarding discrimination against women in medicine and any special plans or programs making it possible for a woman to continue in or return to medicine after leaving the profession to rear a family.

The better trained a woman is and the more advanced her training, the easier it is for her to find a position that is compatible with her home life and the rearing of her children, Dr. Lawrence found. Women without internships are ill-equipped to fill the medical jobs that are now going unfilled. Each year, 20 percent of the residency programs go unfilled, so there is a wide choice of training opportunities for all applicants. The solution, then, is to make these internship and residency programs more accessible to large numbers of women, making it feasible for them to combine this phase of their training with marriage and child rearing.

Dr. Lawrence feels that one way of increasing the supply of doctors to meet the expected shortage in the next decade is to increase the participation of those who have already graduated. Using data on woman graduates not now medically active but still young enough that an investment in their professional rehabilitation would be profitable, she estimates that there is a reservoir of 1,025 women M.D.'s who could be rehabilitated in the next few years. "This would compare with the graduating classes of a dozen medical schools," Dr. Lawrence states.

Married woman physicians are a resource for staffing many of the fields of medicine that do not attract a sufficient number of men.

"The married woman is a 'captive,' " Dr. Lawrence explains. "She must work within her environment and often at a considerably lower salary than if she were unmarried. She has no bargaining power because she cannot pull up stakes and get a more satisfactory contract elsewhere. She must follow her husband, live where he lives, fit her training around his career. It might be pointed out here that marriage for many women is basic to total fulfillment."

A woman, then, finds fulfillment in following her husband and adjusting her career to his. By raising children, a woman doctor gains qualities and attributes that enhance her doctor-patient relationships. A woman who is not compelled to work, who is not the breadwinner, does not compete as intensely as a man to get ahead. She can accept a role in medicine that would be less appealing to a man, can be happy in a position that provides personal satisfaction rather than a large income and recognition.[1]

Dr. Lawrence has dedicated a large portion of her time to exploring and developing programs designed to recruit mother-medics for areas of the profession requiring more practitioners. Her research, findings, and recommendations are detailed in Part III of this book and form the basis for Chapter 18.

In all their career planning, women must develop more open minds, greater flexibility. A woman can bring something different to a field; and while she is making her special contribution to medicine, she should not feel compelled to include all the details of housekeeping in her routine. A woman doctor has something special to give to society; she should accept this opportunity, carve her own niche, and do a good job.

Dr. Lawrence does not have live-in or full-time help, but she does have a dependable baby-sitter, who takes charge of her youngest children when she leaves home, and some cleaning help. She does her own dishes, ironing, and cooking, with assistance from the older children.

When addressing herself to girls planning to enter medical school, Dr. Lawrence says:

"Time and money are the biggest problems, and these can be solved." She does not advise working while in medical school, however.

"I found it better to concentrate all my time on my studies and get top-notch grades. You can do better with scholarships that way." She received scholarship aid through a private foundation and urges girls to consult the various publications available to discover sources of financial aid.

A peek behind the scenes leads to the conclusion that a good sense of humor is essential for leading the double life of doctor and mother of nine. Ruth Lawrence says that often she has to smile when she arrives just in time to present a lecture after giving nine children breakfast, preparing five lunches, making ten beds, and doing three loads of laundry and often after coping with car trouble on the way to the university.

"There are so many little sticky fingers to pass on my way out of the house, I practically have to dress in the garage if I want to make a clean getaway!"

She recalls that her sixth baby had just been born when the date arrived on which she was scheduled to deliver an important lecture. Other faculty members who could have substituted for her were out of town.

"I was still just two days postpartum. I conned the nurses into getting my clothes, and a resident found me a long white coat. Off I went to the classroom, but hospital rules said I was a patient and therefore must go via wheelchair. So I did. I gave the lecture, hopped back into my wheelchair, and arrived back in my room just in time for lunch in bed."

Now there's flexibility!

Many mother-doctors who decide to enter private practice find they can establish an office right at home. This should be kept in mind when the family chooses a house. The doctor (mother) should have a separate wing, preferably with its own entrance, and the mother (doctor) should have child-care help in the household area to cover her absence during office hours.

One woman psychiatrist, the mother of two young sons, wanted to maintain an active but part-time connection with medicine. She established her base of operations in a remodeled porch, and feels that her sylvan setting, on wooded land with a pond, is an asset even though it is not near public transportation. She set her fees so that her patients would benefit from her low overhead, and so that those who had to come from the nearby metropolitan area would be compensated for the extra travel costs.

This woman's avocational interests in nature and writing have resulted in articles for the lay press on teaching children about nature and human values. She is a good example of the way in which a woman with professional training can make use of her education outside her chosen field. Such a mother, intelligent and sensitive, gives the world bright, well-adjusted children and makes additional contributions to the community that are not always directly associated with the practice of medicine.

A husband-and-wife team of general practitioners have devised a way to practice medicine so that the wife can fulfill her career ambitions without conflict in their marriage. The husband takes all nighttime emergency calls, and the wife handles the early-morning office hours. Then the husband handles the late-afternoon office hours, so that the wife can be at home when the children return from school and can prepare the family dinner.

As the husband put it: "This works!"

Dr. Margaret J. Giannini is professor of pediatrics and director of the Center for Mental Retardation of New York Medical College, in New York City. She is the wife of a distinguished obstetrician and gynecologist, Dr. Louis J. Salerno, who is chief of obstetric and gynecological services at Flower and Fifth Avenue Hospitals, and the mother of four sons (ages eighteen, fourteen, twelve, and ten), who have become involved in serving others through the example of her dedication to the mentally retarded. The center, opened eighteen years ago at the Flower and Fifth Avenue Hospitals of New York Medical College, is not only the oldest and largest of its kind, but is a pacesetter in methods. Begun at the request of a group of parents of retarded children, it was the first to stress a multidisciplinary approach to retardation combining diagnosis, treatment, rehabilitation, teaching, and research.

"Even a normal person degenerates in an institution," Dr. Giannini points out. "There may not be a cure for these children yet, but there's always hope. They can be helped to lead happy, useful lives. Many of the clinic's patients are now self-supporting."

There were no precedents for such a clinic; so Dr. Giannini developed the multidisciplinary attack on mental retardation and fostered research into its causes. She began with three part-time pediatricians and seventeen volunteers, most of them also part time. The clinic is for the parents as well as the child, for Dr. Giannini firmly believes that, because of the nature of the child's affliction, the parents, too, need counseling and treatment. The total program eventually helps the child realize his highest level of development.

Dr. Giannini married Dr. Salerno upon completion of her residency. Their children began arriving two years after she had started her medical practice.

Because of her commitments as mother, doctor, and director of the Mental Retardation Center, Dr. Giannini admits to being compulsive about time—her most precious commodity.

"Time must not be wasted; it must be used for a purpose. I must not sacrifice any area of my responsibility. If there is an existing conflict, it is that there are not as many hours in the day as there are things I would like to do."

She recalls with humor one logjam of activities that taxed even her capacity for structuring time. Her ten-year-old son, Louis, was scheduled to give a piano recital at his school, St. David's, in Manhattan, the same day as she was to be the guest speaker at a luncheon for government dignitaries.

"There were important visitors from Washington, plus the usual pressure of clinic business. When the door had closed on the VIP's, I picked up my purse and told my secretary I'd be at St. David's School."

Her secretary replied, "I can almost see that inside your head you have a million orderly compartments, all separately filed and cross-indexed, with a built-in timer. Nothing ever gets lost."

"The recital was good," Dr. Giannini remembers fondly. "Louis beamed from the stage at me, and I beamed back. Being there was as important as anything I had done that day."

Dr. Giannini surmounts the problems of a working mother by eliminating them. She feels that children's emotional needs can be satisfied in less than twenty-four hours a day. "I can cluck in sympathy over a scraped knee or an adolescent pimple just like anyone else," she says, "and supply a bandage as well as a kiss."

Her conviction is that you must give children your completely undivided attention when you are with them. "Listening to the boys is an education in itself. And *I do listen,* and they know that I do, so they are able to talk freely," she says.

"I have never broken a promise to them—I feel very strongly about that . . . The boys know that they will always receive my attention when it really counts. They understand that I have another important side to my life, just as they do."

Instead of trying to compete with this other life, these perceptive youngsters involve themselves in it.

Twelve-year-old Justin, in the eighth grade at St. David's, suggested that the boys in his class form a "buddy system" to work with the mentally retarded boys at the center. The class approved the project, and Justin and his teacher broached the subject to Dr. Giannini.

"I had mixed feelings when the experiment started," Dr. Giannini admits. "Both my husband and I were concerned that the students were too young to work effectively with the retarded boys."

The results have melted away those original doubts, and the efforts of the St. David's boys have met with enthusiasm from parents, staff members, and the boys at the center.

Every Thursday afternoon, the eighth-graders help the retarded boys to learn simple games, play cooperatively, and make friends. So far as the center's staff knows, it is the first such experiment anywhere.

"A retarded child is often acutely lonely," Dr. Giannini says thoughtfully. "His difficulty in communicating severely hinders his contacts and friendships with other children. Although retarded children can learn to develop their limited abilities through the kind of therapy and special training available at the center, this important area of their lives remains untouched."

It was in the area of promoting friendship, of teaching an attitude of give-and-take, that Justin and his classmates were able to help the retarded youngsters the most. The boys from St. David's were sympathetic from the start, and very soon the children found points of common interest. The center's children clearly enjoyed the new attention. Although parties tended to be somewhat formal at first, they soon warmed up. Now, in their excitement over toy cars, paint pots, and refreshments, the two groups of boys often forget their differing circumstances. The discovery of things in common is, to the center's staff, one of the most rewarding aspects of the sessions.

Those who accuse physician-mothers of decreasing their contributions to medicine when they spend time with their children would do well to examine the beneficial effects such dedicated women have on their families and on the community. In 1968, Dr. Giannini was one of fifty women interested in child health who were invited to luncheon at the White House by Mrs. Lyndon Johnson. Dr. Giannini is a member of the Mayor's Committee on Retardation, working in the New York Metropolitan area to coordinate existing resources for the retarded and to develop a complete range of essential programs in each of the city's boroughs.

All these activities would not be possible without reliable household help, Dr. Giannini emphasizes. Since she and her husband both are physicians, they are aware of their dual professional and family responsibilities. Although the family has never employed sleep-in help, a full-time governess cared for the children throughout their early years and still baby-sits with the younger boys when needed. A five-day-a-week housekeeper maintains the home and cooks the meals. "Weekends, I am the sole housekeeper, and I do enjoy my domesticity," says Dr. Giannini.

Because they have sufficient help, the two doctors are free to devote their leisure time exclusively to the children and each other.

"My husband and I never take a separate vacation; we only take family holidays. In the Bahamas during Easter week we all tried skin diving. We also go swimming, golfing, and bowling together, and when the weather is right we enjoy outdoor barbecues. In the winter, we take an occasional ski weekend. Birthdays are always festive occasions. We have some 'musicales' at home, and the boys get 'A' for effort if not perfection."

There are family rules, but both parents work toward maintaining a healthy balance between discipline and freedom. The three younger boys freely discuss with their mother whatever perplexes them, and she tries to guide them in reaching their own solutions. The oldest boy, Robert, is away at school, but Dr. Giannini confesses that, when he is at home and goes out for an evening, she likes to wait up for him. It gives them both an opportunity to spend some special time together. "Robert is the most reticent of my sons, and it is in those quiet moments that he opens up, and we sit and chat about all sorts of things."

Dr. Giannini believes that the maternal-medical combination is a natural one, and that the two careers can be equally fulfilling. To illustrate this belief, she relates the following incident that took place in her office.

One of her male colleagues was introducing her to a fashionable career woman who had an important position in public relations.

"This is Dr. Giannini," he said, "the director of our center." Smiling, he picked up the framed family portrait from her desk and added, "but she's a woman first."

"I suppose I like that," Dr. Giannini smiles.

Notes to Chapter Four

1. Ruth Anderson Lawrence, M.D., "The Training of Women Physicians," presented at Josiah Macy, Jr., Foundation conference on *Women for Medicine,* Dedham, Mass., October, 1966.

Chapter Five

MEDICAL CAREERS ESPECIALLY SUITED FOR MARRIED WOMEN

Few girls know how varied are their career choices in medicine. The traditional fields that most people consider ideal for woman physicians, such as private practice in pediatrics or obstetrics, are so demanding on their time that they really are not the most suitable. As Dr. Ruth Lawrence emphasizes, young women contemplating medicine must be informed about careers that will complement, rather than compete with, family life. Many of the women now in such paramedical fields as nursing and medical technology are apostates who have decided the M.D. is out of reach.

But opportunity for women in medicine decidedly does exist. The challenge is to determine in what areas—of the profession and, geographically, of the nation—they can be most successful. In seeking admittance to medical school, in postgraduate experience, and in practice, a woman should consider how great the need is for the particular career or specialty she wishes to pursue. By contacting local medical societies, reading health and manpower source studies, and questioning physicians and teachers, a young woman contemplating medicine can learn which localities need her the most.

The American Medical Association publishes annually a book presenting data on the distribution of physicians in the United States. The 1967 edition, available from the AMA at $2.40 per copy, is entitled *Distribution of Physicians, Hospitals, and Hospital Beds in the U.S., Regional, State, County, Metropolitan Area.* It provides information on the geographic distribution of medical practice in the United States and its possessions.

Listings include physicians employed by the federal government distributed by census region and division, specialty, activity, and branch of service. Activity and specialty data on nonfederal physicians are given by region, division, state, county, and metropolitan areas.

The AMA believes that the 219 Standard Metropolitan Statistical Areas (SMSA's) and 81 Potential SMSA's are deserving of special attention because of the increased urbanization of the United States: "The 300 SMSA's contain 85.2 percent of the nonfederal physicians in the United States and possessions. Physicians in medical, surgical, and other specialties located in metropolitan areas constitute larger percentages than those in general practice." The heavy concentration of health care services in large metropolitan areas is readily apparent, as are similarly heavy concentrations of medical schools and pharmaceutical companies.[1]

On the county level (nonfederal physicians only), the thirty-four AMA-recognized specialties are grouped into four categories; general practice, medical specialties, surgical specialties, and other specialties. In addition, hospital, income, and resident population data are supplied for each county.

The physician-population ratio is highest in the Northeast and, according to the United States Public Health Service,[2] lowest in the South. A woman establishing a practice in an area with a shortage of doctors could set her own precedents and control her work load at the outset. For example, the idea of two or three mother-doctors sharing a pediatric practice would be readily accepted in a community where pediatricians were urgently needed.

Predictability of working hours is the most important factor in maintaining a harmonious balance between the practice of medicine and running a home. As one doctor put it: "It takes a very unusual man to put up with a doctor-wife. If she had to take night calls, most men would not like it."

While there are many examples of women successfully balancing a private practice and a home and family, there is a wide variety of other career opportunities that can be pursued during the busy years of early marriage, when the babies are arriving and the children are too young for school. This chapter will explore a number of these medical careers that mix well with marriage.

Academic Medicine

Here is one area where women will get almost no opposition from men in medicine.

"The idea of academic medicine as a career for women is an excellent one," Dr. James Bartlett, of the University of Rochester, contends. "There are many possibilities for working out a variety of assignments, and teaching is clearly one of the most vital needs. There are a number of women now on our own faculty, and their contributions are major ones."

"Women do have a contribution to make in academic medicine," states Dr. George Lewis, associate dean at the University of Miami School of Medicine (Florida). "In order to expand medical facilities and train more students, we must first have more teachers. The trouble with women entering medicine is that the traditional career for a woman in our society is to get married and have a family. I think the place where women can best fit into the profession is in areas in which physicians are needed but which have fixed working hours—not private practice."

Dr. Libby Connor, clinical instructor in medicine at the University of Miami's medical school, agrees, with one important reservation:

"Academic medicine offers predictable hours—you do have some time for your family. However, you can't really say one area of medicine is best for women, for if someone goes into medicine she has certain reasons; you have to do what you want to do. If you like to teach, academic medicine is ideal; if not, you don't belong there."

Dr. Connor thinks that any woman who really wants to go into medicine should be encouraged, but cautions that it is not the right career for everyone. "Young girls like the glamour associated with the hospital. It is a lot of work just to have someone call you 'doctor.' "

She also emphasizes that many girls don't appreciate how rapidly medicine is changing and that they can't afford to lose touch. This is a major consideration for a girl; she is going to have to pursue her profession part-time. A woman can leave almost any other career and come back to it after her children are grown. The woman doctor can't—and medical schools want young people who will use their training for many years.

Dr. Connor teaches one sophomore course in preventive medicine, but most of her teaching is done in the clinical years. She and other members of the clinical staff in the department of medicine alternate making rounds and teaching the ward teams. She says that even when she is on ward duty it is a rare night when she has to return to the hospital to see an acutely ill patient.

"Patients admitted to this ward—infectious disease—I see immediately. The house staff attends to their diagnosis and treatment. Things are handled very well within my teaching hours. If I am not in the hospital, one of the interns or residents sees the new cases. The interns can check with me by phone or with one of the faculty members who are always within the hospital. The ward teams are always supervised."

Residents, Dr. Connor points out, can take a great deal of the night-call burden from faculty members. While many people erroneously regard a resident as a student because he is still in a learning situation, this is not the case. "The resident is qualified to be out in practice by himself. He is in no way only a student."

Until the arrival of her first baby, now a handsome six-month-old son smiling out from a picture on her desk, Dr. Connor did all her own housework. Since then, she has had a girl in one day a week to iron and to clean her floors—"and that's about it; I do my own cooking."

As for child care during the hours she is out of the home: "I am fortunate in having a neighbor who takes care of the baby. A major consideration is having someone to be near the baby and love him like her own. If you have this mother figure to take over in your absence, you are most fortunate and can have children during these busy years. I am still breast-feeding my son after six months, which is probably longer than most nonworking mothers do."

Libby Connor believes she was particularly fortunate in the well-ordered way she was able to prepare for her career. Hers is probably the ideal schedule for a girl entering medicine, and the best carried out of any mother-doctor interviewed for this book. As she is an only child, her father could finance her medical education at Cornell. She realizes how lucky she was that there were no brothers or sisters to be sent to college while she was in medical school.

"I married after both my internship and residency were complete. I think this is ideal—of course, it depends on when you meet the right man!"

Many more clinical teachers of medicine are needed, and better salaries will attract them. "Pay for clinical teachers is not satisfactory," Dr. Connor says. "In academic medicine, if you wish to make a living you almost have to do research. To get ahead at all in this area, basic laboratory research has to be done to some degree."

In this regard, the medical schools are creating their own conundrum. "So long as medical schools are 'poor,' they are going to accept the young research men who bring in the grants." The more emphasis there is on research, and on research as the criterion for advancement in academic medicine, the less emphasis on the importance of teaching medical students. Hence, the medical teacher shortage.

Another means of entering academic medicine is through attainment of the Ph.D. degree in the basic medical sciences. Many faculty members of medical schools are not physicians, but hold doctorates in fields such as chemistry, microbiology, pharmacology, and radiology. They lecture mainly in the preclinical years and also engage in laboratory research.

The *Journal of the American Medical Association* states: "Graduate programs in the basic medical sciences are recognized as an important source of future faculty members for the medical school basic science departments and, to a lesser extent, for the clinical departments. Consequently, the number of graduate students is directly relevant to the problem of meeting manpower needs." [3]

"My fun is the students," Dr. Connor smiles. "I enjoy them. If we don't concentrate on teaching as the primary concern, we then forget what the medical school is for."

Academic medicine has everything going for it as the career choice of the woman physician. She can practice medicine in the teaching hospital and maintain contact with patients, utilizing her special skills and compassionate nature. She has the opportunity for creative involvement in laboratory research and for being in constant touch with the latest developments in her field. She has the stimulation of working with each new class of students, their questions and their learning process continually augmenting her own. She has the satisfaction of entering a field in which her skills are urgently needed, in which a personnel shortage is felt in every part of the United States. The regular hours and variety of teaching schedules available, both full- and part-time, combine well with marriage and a family.

Also important is the woman medical academician's total acceptance by her male colleagues. "I have never felt any discrimination at any point in my career because I was a woman," Dr. Connor says. "I have had people tell me that they had been prepared not to like working under me because I was a woman, but I was not aware of it at the time they were on my service."

Dr. Connor grinned mischievously, tossed back her long blonde hair, and offered the following rejoinder for the use of any young woman who encounters the mother-stay-out-of-medicine attitude:

"The only time any faculty member ever mentioned anything to me about being a woman at any time in my career was when I was looking at internships. An old codger asked me why they should take me when I would lose ten years, at least part-time away from the profession, as a mother raising a family. I retorted that the life expectancy of a woman is at least ten years longer than that of a man!"

Administration

Medical administration offers work in the business side of the profession to the organization-minded woman. Hospitals, pharmaceutical laboratories, universities, research centers, volunteer organizations, school health programs, private industry, labor unions, and the federal, state, and local governments all require medical doctors with business acumen to plan, direct, and carry out their programs.

A few courses in business administration are worth including in your premedical undergraduate study if such a career appeals to you. The ability to plan programs and see them through to completion should be part of your makeup. A most important consideration for you as a woman is that your talents can be utilized during regular business hours. Although some doctors will feel regret at the loss of patient contact, medical administrators must remember that they still have the challenge of working with people in their capacity as supervisors.

The medical administrator often designs and directs programs to put the latest developments in medicine into practice. Any research in new techniques, treatments, drugs, and so on would be pointless if these advances were not translated into patient care. You can direct area-wide planning for total patient care, coordinate the activities of agencies and services, teach preventive medicine, or work in one of the many phases of public health. There is a wide choice in assignments, a continuing demand for competent personnel, and great flexibility in the number of hours you can choose to devote to this career.

Anesthesiology

Anesthesiology ranks fourth as a specialty choice for woman physicians.[4]

Dr. Albert Betcher of the American Society of Anesthesiologists states that "anesthesiology ranks high [as a career choice] because it is an institutional practice requiring no expenditure for office or equipment, because the hours of elective surgery are between 8:00 A.M. and 5:00 P.M., and because in some hospitals with a large number of anesthesiologists on the staff arrangements can be made for part-time appointments. Unlike specialties in which return visits to the same physician are a must, in this one most contacts with a patient begin with the preanesthetic visit and are concluded with the postoperative visit." [5]

The length of residency is either two or three years, and a physician can elect either of two plans of training (plus practice time) in order to be eligible for certification by the American Board of Anesthesiology.

The board recognizes that married woman physicians are most likely to have children during the time they are in their residency training. To insure that mother-physicians will not drop out of their postgraduate training programs, the board will, in individual cases, grant credit for part-time training in an approved hospital. In some cases, two women might share one slot for residency training, giving full coverage to the hospital and receiving proportional credit for the actual time spent. Part-time duty will, of course, prolong the time needed to obtain accreditation.

The anesthesiologist does not just administer anesthetic agents. In addition to knowing the technical methods of anesthesia, he must have a thorough knowledge of the management of patients undergoing all types of surgery. He must also have a thorough understanding of the body processes and organ functions. It is not enough to know the properties of various drugs; the anesthesiologist must understand the mechanisms by which the drugs produce their effects. And he should be experienced in related fields, such as diagnostic and therapeutic nerve blocks, problems in resuscitation and airway management, problems in sedation, inhalation therapy, and the technique of bronchoscopy.

In addition, the anesthesiologist participates in the care of patients outside the operating room. He is first of all a physician, and as such must be familiar with the fundamental aspects of the disorders affecting his patients and with the impact therapy may have on them, so that he can adjust his management of the anesthesia. He participates in the preanesthetic preparation and evaluation of the patient as well as in the postanesthetic and postoperative care.[6]

Dentistry

Rarely does a girl dream of becoming a dentist, yet this profession has ample room for her. The nation's supply of dentists has been declining for years in relation to population. According to the American Dental Association,[7] only one out of every hundred practicing dentists in the United States is a woman. In dentistry, as in medicine, America has a minute percentage of women compared to foreign countries: 80 percent of the dentists in Russia, Finland, and Lithuania are women, 50 percent in Greece, 23 to 30 percent in France and the Scandinavian countries. Our 1 percent is the smallest proportion of women dentists of any nation in the Western Hemisphere.

Dentistry offers women many benefits. Dental practice is independent; a woman can adjust her hours to suit her changing family needs. When the children are young, she can practice part-time or limit herself to group practice or practice in a clinic. As the youngsters grow, she can expand her hours to include the time they are in school, and when they are grown she will have an established full-time profession. Many dentists have their offices in their homes— an ideal situation for the woman wishing to combine dentistry with household duties.

The experience and understanding a mother can bring to the specialty of pedodontics—children's dentistry—are a valuable asset in the handling of young patients. A mother is also more aware of other parents' anxiety for their children, and her empathy with parental concern could easily win their confidence.

Predental study (discussed below) is shorter than premed and offers a wider choice of curricula, although about 50 percent of the students entering dental school choose to earn the B.A. degree first. Dental education is less costly than medical education. The average cost to a state resident in a state-supported dental school is about twelve hundred dollars a year, including tuition; for nonresidents, it is about seventeen hundred dollars. There are many sources of financial assistance for dental students.

A woman's future in dentistry is secure, the gap between the number of dentists graduated each year and the number needed has created a shortage that will extend for decades. Practicing dentists earn an average of nineteen thousand dollars *net* annual income. A woman with a D.D.S. is welcome in any country of the world, as every observant traveler will confirm. Dentistry offers the personal reward of extending a needed service to suffering patients. As the American Dental Association states:

"Most important, dentistry is an extremely rewarding profession, as dentists perform truly humanitarian services—relieving pain, correcting oral problems, and preventing oral disease." [8]

Careers in Dentistry. General dentistry can be practiced privately, in clinics, in the armed forces, and in many agencies of government, including public health services. Administrative careers are also open to dentists in government, industry, and private organizations.

There are eight areas of specialization in dentistry. Children's dentistry (pedodontics) attracts the greatest number of women. So great is the attraction of this specialty, in fact, that the dental association of one large metropolitan area reports that all of its woman dentists limit their practice to children.

The other specialties are orthodontics, the treatment and correction of irregularities of the teeth, especially by mechanical aids (braces); periodontics, the treatment of gum diseases; oral surgery; endodontics, the preservation of dead teeth through special therapy; public health; prosthodontics, the care of denture patients; and oral pathology, the study of the origin of oral disease. This last area offers opportunities for research in the causes and therapeutics of oral disease.

Other areas of dental research needing intelligent investigation are those of congenital defects, such as cleft palate and cleft lip; of a cure for oral cancer; and of dental decay.

Academic dentistry offers all the advantages of academic medicine. There is a continuing need for teachers to educate future dentists.

Requirements for Admission to Dental School. The American Dental Association lists the following basic requirements for students wishing to gain admission to dental school: [9]

1. A minimum of two years of college, preferably in a liberal arts curriculum. You must have completed one year each of biology, chemistry, and physics, and one year of English. An additional half year of organic chemistry is also required.

2. You must take the Dental Aptitude Test, which measures

your potential as a dental student and as a practicing dentist. This test measures intellectual and manual aptitudes, not specific achievement. You should have completed at least one year of college and your course requirements in biology and chemistry before taking the test, but no other special preparation is necessary.

The Council on Dental Education of the American Dental Association (211 East Chicago Avenue, Chicago, Illinois 60611) offers a free booklet, *Dental Aptitude Testing Program,* that gives further details. Specific dates and places for taking the aptitude test can be obtained from any dental school.

3. An application form from the dental school of your choice must be submitted at least one year in advance of your intended entrance into that school. High school and college transcripts must also be submitted, along with the appropriate letters of recommendation.

If you will require financial assistance during dental study, write to the dental school you plan to attend, since all financial aid is administered by the individual school. Specific information on loans and scholarships available through that particular school will be given to you by the office of financial aid.

Once accepted by a dental school, you will begin a four-year program of intensive study in both the science and the art of dentistry. You will be qualified to enter general practice immediately upon graduation, without further internship. However, if you intend to specialize, you will be required to spend two or more years of postgraduate study after dental school in a hospital or educational institution.

An excellent booklet, *Admission Requirements of American Dental Schools,* gives general information on all dental schools in the United States and Canada, including tuition and living costs, educational requirements for admission, and sources of financial aid. It is available at two dollars per copy from: American Association of Dental Schools, 211 East Chicago Avenue, Chicago, Illinois 60611.

Two other publications that the prospective dental student may find helpful are *Careers in Dentistry,* available without charge from the Council on Dental Education, American Dental Association, 211 East Chicago Avenue, Chicago, Illinois 60611, and *Frontiers of Dental Science,* available at fifty cents per copy from the American Dental Association.

Dermatology

The specialty of dermatology offers the possibility of combining a practice in clinical medicine with a career in research, or the option of emphasizing one or the other. This field has the advantage that there are never any emergency calls, and the office hours of the practicing specialist can be easily adjusted to a schedule compatible with the needs of family life.

A wider variety of background study and experience is applicable to dermatology than to many other specialties. Training in such fields as biochemistry, physics, cellular pathology, microbiology, genetics, and statistics probably is more readily utilizable in dermatology than in almost any other medical specialty. A physician practicing in clinical dermatology can engage concurrently in research projects concerned with the skin; furthermore, he can do without much of the highly specialized and expensive technical equipment and the elaborate facilities required in many other medical disciplines.

Residencies, fellowship programs, and postgraduate training are available throughout the country. In government programs and the armed forces, study can be carried on overseas. To gain experience in this field, the physician is not restricted to one geographical area or to one locality with a concentration of specialized equipment and facilities.

In clinical medicine, dermatology is valuable in diagnosis not only of diseases of the skin itself, but of allergic diseases, diphtheria, tuberculosis, and many other maladies that seem removed from cutaneous involvement. In research, a dermatologist can explore a fascinating variety of subjects, from the familiar responses to emotional stimuli, such as blushing, goose pimples, and sweating, to the most complex biochemical reactions. Study of the skin leads to discoveries about its own functions and an understanding of other body tissues.

Ophthalmology

The ophthalmologist is a physician specializing in the study and treatment of defects and diseases of the eye. After completing studies for the M.D. and serving an internship, the future ophthalmologist must serve a residency of three years, which includes special training in the eye and the visual system plus experience in closely related fields of medicine and surgery.

The woman ophthalmologist will find that here, too, the scope of her practice can be adjusted to her changing family needs. Her time can be divided among private practice, a hospital appointment, surgery, and full-time research, or combinations of these that suit her schedule at a particular stage of her career. Most of the work can be handled by appointment, and emergencies are comparatively rare—depending mainly on the percentage of surgical cases. Part-time work can be arranged through hospitals and institutions, or by serving a few days per week in a school, an industrial concern, or a business firm.

The equipment required to practice ophthalmology is expensive. For this reason, an institutional appointment or partnership practice is a good choice for a woman who may not wish to take on the sole responsibility for purchasing a large amount of special apparatus.

One woman ophthalmologist has pointed out, in the *Journal of the American Medical Women's Association,* that the delicacy of the eye and the small size of the organ seem to suit a woman's capacity for detailed work and for accuracy and attention. Some of the aspects of eye surgery are retinal surgery and correction of detached retinas, corneal transplants, cataract removal, muscle surgery, and reconstruction of the eyelid.

The eye is also an indicator of general health, reflecting symptoms of many types of physical disorders and emotional fatigue. For this reason, it is a constant challenge to the diagnostician who is aware that he is treating the entire patient, not an isolated organ.

The specialty board in ophthalmology does not approve extended or part-time residencies. However, the rare possibility exists of receiving a preceptorship in the private office of a staff member in ophthalmology. This can give a woman an added chance to work out scheduling that fits her needs, although it is not considered the most desirable means of gaining training.[10]

Opportunities in research in this field are extensive. They combine regularity of work hours with patient contact and the challenge of a rapidly expanding body of specialized knowledge. A few of the fascinating possibilities for investigation by curious and dedicated ophthalmologists are congenital defects of the eye, psychosomatic ophthalmology, the application of research findings to reading difficulties in children, and the effect of poor vision on an individual's earning capacity.

Psychiatry

A psychiatrist is a physician (M.D.) who deals specifically with the prevention, diagnosis, and treatment of mental disorders. This specialty requires completion of the hospital internship and then a three-year residency in an approved hospital or agency concerned with the diagnosis and treatment of mental and emotional disorders. The subspecialty of child psychiatry requires an additional two-year residency plus certification in psychiatry.

After completion of the residency, at least two years of additional professional experience must be acquired before a physician can take the examination for certification by the American Board of Psychiatry and Neurology.[11]

The specialty of psychiatry offers a wide range of areas for practice and considerable leeway in the amount of time the woman doctor can devote to the profession at any period of her life. Mental retardation, alcoholism, delinquency, geriatrics, and preventive psychiatry are only a few of the fields in which part-time jobs, full-time appointments, research, and private practice are available. The demand for qualified psychiatrists far exceeds the supply, and this is one medical specialty that has been actively recruiting women for some time.

Among the settings in which psychiatrists work are mental hospitals, psychiatric sections of general hospitals, community mental health centers, and outpatient clinics. Industrial psychiatry, public health, student health, rehabilitation, and legal psychiatry are other areas of interest, and these can often be combined with private practice.

The psychiatrist identifies the patient's individual problems, administers or prescribes appropriate therapies, and, in general, directs or gives the kind of care and treatment needed. Some psychiatrists also are trained in psychoanalysis, a special form of psychotherapy in which the patient is helped to discover and understand the unconscious, deeply buried causes of his emotional problems. Such psychiatrists are called psychoanalysts.

Dr. Ruth Lawrence, in her study on the training of woman physicians (*see* Chapter 4), discovered that part-time work was not difficult to find in psychiatry.

"The department chairmen were more sympathetic to the mother-doctor and her dual responsibilities. Women trained in this area were keeping active and felt as if they were getting a fair shake. Many felt that child psychiatry was the ideal spot for the mother-doctor. In psychiatry, it was felt, there is a great interest in attracting candidates for training who have satisfying personal lives and who are relatively free of debilitating emotional conflicts." [12]

Psychiatry is the first medical specialty to tailor a graduate training program to the dual commitments of the woman physician with a family who wishes to continue her professional training. A great effort is being made by administrators in this field to eliminate the stigma attached to woman psychiatrists because they occasionally must request a little time off to cope with a family emergency. A detailed study of the residency program in psychiatry for mother-doctors at New York Medical College is presented in Part III.

Pathology

This field is rapidly gaining popularity with women in medicine and now ranks fifth as their specialty choice. [13] Pathology offers the opportunity to pursue research and engage in diagnosis, plus the satisfaction afforded by productive use of analytic techniques—all within regular business hours and an established daily routine.

The pathologist examines specimens of diseased tissues, with the naked eye and microscopically, to determine the nature and cause of the disease affecting the patient. He reads biopsies—tissues removed from patients for diagnosis—to determine, usually, if a tumor or growth is malignant and further surgical procedures are called for. He examines frozen sections in emergency cases in which a patient is in surgery and the surgeon requires immediate verification of an affected tissue. In such a case, a specimen is removed, quick-frozen, and prepared on slides; the pathologist examines these and reports his findings while the surgery is in progress.

The pathologist working at a teaching hospital usually has an appointment to the clinical faculty. He does some lecturing at the medical school, reviews cases with residents, and teaches, in small lecture groups, students and interns assigned to the service.

After receiving his M.D. and completing internship, the physician planning to specialize in pathology must take a four-year residency to become board-certified in both clinical and anatomic pathology.

The field of clinical pathology includes chemical pathology, the chemical study of body fluids, in which examination is made of the changes in these fluids caused by disease; hematology, the microscopic and chemical study of the cellular components of the blood, i.e., the red and white cells, the platelets, and the factors that make blood clot; and microbiology, the study of microorganisms, such as bacteria, viruses, and fungi.

Anatomic pathology includes the microscopic study of tissues, mainly tumors (i.e., cancer) that are removed during surgery; the study of tissues in the postmortem room to observe what changes have been produced by disease; and cytology, the microscopic study, to observe any abnormal growth, of cells that have been shed from various body surfaces.

To be certified in either clinical or anatomic pathology, a three-year residency is required. If certified in only one field, you could practice only in a large hospital where many pathologists are employed, each devoting all his time to one segment of the specialty. In smaller hospitals and in laboratories, the pathologist would have to be responsible for the whole spectrum of pathologic studies.

Even in a large hospital, the department chairman or laboratory director must be certified in both fields, because he would be in charge of both divisions. In practice, most pathologists are certified in both. If you aspire to direct a laboratory, you would be limited by certification in one field only.

Training and practice in pathology are not as demanding on a woman's time as many other specialties. Female pathologists think it is an ideal career for a woman who likes the field and has a genuine interest in it.

"If you are interested in medicine, [as a pathologist] you are *doing* medicine and at the same time have a regular schedule," said one. "But I did not choose the field because of the hours or any other specific advantage," she hastened to add. "I think it is an important part of medicine and planned my entrance into the field right from the beginning of my studies. I wanted to do some useful work with results that I could see applied directly to the patients."

Once a woman has earned her M.D. and completed her internship, residency in pathology is quite compatible with the demands of family life. She works in the hospital from 8:00 A.M. until about 4:30 P.M., with one or two nights a week on call. Most emergency calls are completed before midnight. "You get some frozen sections up until 10 or 11 P.M., and sometimes have to perform an autopsy in late evening," said a woman pathologist, "but there is rarely a middle-of-the-night call as in many of the other services. I never had to sleep at the hospital on my call nights."

After training is completed, there often is little or no night work.

The frequency of night calls or emergency work depends on the type of hospital in which you work. Some, particularly the smaller institutions, have many night calls. Larger hospitals usually have night calls assigned to particular personnel, often the senior residents in pathology. If a surgeon is operating in the middle of the night and encounters a tumor that he cannot immediately identify, the first thing he does is call in a pathologist to make a frozen section. Pathologists are not guaranteed that there will never be night emergencies.

Mother-pathologists recommend working in a hospital or institution rather than in private practice, because the latter is more time-consuming. A woman pathologist can establish her own laboratory, particularly in a locality that has no large hospitals with extensive laboratory facilities. A thriving practice can be built by serving two or three small hospitals, doing their laboratory pathological work and autopsies. If you have your own lab, you make more money, but such ownership makes additional demands on you. A compromise possibility would be an affiliation or partnership in such an endeavor.

Drawbacks? "Well, if a woman does not like to work with autopsy material, this would not be the place for her," laughed one young resident. "But it has never bothered me. I like laboratory work and I find the job fascinating. The most important thing is to know what you want in life—in any field."

Pediatrics

This is one specialty that needs no tub-thumping to attract female physicians to its ranks. Pediatrics is the foremost specialty choice of women.[14] As more than one doctor has pointed out, however, it is not necessarily the ideal career for the woman with a family, because the demands made on her time and energies by a pediatric practice often can run round the clock.

There are ways to control the amount of time devoted to a career in pediatrics. Both Dr. Ruth Lawrence and Dr. Margaret Giannini, featured in Chapter 4, are involved in the institutional practice and teaching of their specialty. For the individual desiring private practice, a group or partnership practice in which emergency calls are shared is another option.

Women are attracted to this specialty for the obvious reason that nature has cast them in the mother's role, and therefore this area is one where women traditionally have been accepted and have felt welcome. Whether or not they are mothers, women often possess an empathy with children that men seem to lack. As one male physician pointed out:

"A child left alone in a hospital may scream in fright when a male doctor approaches him. When he hears a woman's voice, it quiets him. The smaller children in particular seem more relaxed with a female pediatrician."

A special relationship frequently develops between the parents of the sick child and a mother-pediatrician. No one understands better than a mother the anguish parents suffer when their child is seriously ill.

Dr. Giannini, herself a pediatrician, knows this feeling well: "I am alert to a serious illness or a childhood disease in my own children, but like any other doctor, or any other mother, I call in another physician to treat my children—and stand by, I suppose like any other mother, with an affirmative smile while mentally wringing my hands."

The pediatrician specializes in the growth and development of the child from birth to adolescence. The duration of residency for pediatrics is two years. The pediatrician must be trained in general medical pediatrics plus care of newborn infants, preventive pediatrics, nutritional disorders, contagious diseases, and neurological disorders. A wide range of experience is gained from working at outpatient clinics in the teaching hospital and in well-baby clinics and centers for the mentally deficient.

The primary reason for including pediatrics in this chapter is the attitude of the profession toward woman's role in this specialty. Pediatrics is one of the two specialties (the other is psychiatry) where women with family commitments are able to make special arrangements for continuing work or returning to the field. Part-time work is not difficult to find, and department chairmen of pediatrics are sympathetic to the dual roles of mother-physicians and their resulting responsibilities.[15] The specialty board occasionally will permit part-time training, on an individual basis. It is up to the individual to initiate a request for such consideration.

Public Health

The field of public health is so vast and the need for personnel so great that any interested woman physician can find her niche in this specialty and make her contribution. A young, single woman may want to take an overseas assignment before marriage, for instance, and after marriage work part-time as a school physician while raising her children. Whatever her work needs, full-time employment or only a few hours a week, the public health services have a place for the woman doctor. Whether her area of interest is direct medical service, research, training programs, or health education, she can readily practice her specialty. Public health permits participation by doctors with a wide variety of medical backgrounds. One can either specialize directly in the public health field or apply to it the training gained from another specialty.

Formal training for the public health career includes a year in a school of public health, leading to a degree of master of public health.[16] Those expecting to enter the research and education areas of public health find it advisable to obtain the advanced degree of doctor of public health. Short-term training institutes, courses, and seminars also are available to physicians interested in this career.

The United States Public Health Service administers a public health traineeship program for which members of all the health professions are eligible. On receipt of a medical degree, a physician can apply for a traineeship. Applicants also must have been accepted by the training institution of their choice for the proposed program of study.

Institutions offering approved residency programs in general preventive medicine and in preventive medicine-public health are now eligible, under the public health traineeship program, to apply for grants for specific individuals who have been tentatively accepted for those programs. To get further information, write to:

Training Resources Branch
Division of Community Health Services
Public Health Service
U. S. Department of Health, Education, and Welfare
Washington, D. C. 20201

Careers in the Federal Public Health Service. The U. S. Public Health Service is the major federal agency responsible for protecting and advancing the health of the nation. The service defines its goals as follows: "The health programs are designed to protect citizens against illness and disease; guard against importation of disease; expand health facilities and services; create a more healthful environment; conduct research into major health problems; increase knowledge of the cause, treatment, control, and/or prevention of all major diseases of humanity; further improve and prolong human life." [17]

To fulfill these health-promoting responsibilities, the service operates a far-reaching system of programs stretching across the nation and around the world, and including 350 professional and supporting activities in health and health-related programs; a great network of facilities, including 16 hospitals, 43 Indian hospitals, 135 outpatient clinics, 100 field stations, and 380 quarantine stations in the United States and abroad; and the world-famed National Institutes of Health research facilities.

The U. S. Public Health Service offers everything from the security of regular hours in stateside positions to the challenge of rotating assignments overseas. This is a career service that welcomes women in medicine with open arms. Government service for doctors also includes the armed forces, the Veterans Administration, the Peace Corps, and the Head Start programs.

Career opportunities include:

Medicine: clinical research, direct and indirect medical care, administration.

Science and research: physics, biology, genetics, radiology, air pollution, water pollution, pharmacology.

Dentistry: clinical, research, public health, and administration.

Epidemiology: clinical, research, public health.

PHS conducts research into nearly every problem area in the health field. It assists states and communities through grants, consultation, and technical assistance and exerts a leading role in national and international health affairs. Detailed information on entry into the Public Health Service is available from:

Surgeon General
Public Health Service
U. S. Department of Health, Education, and Welfare
Washington, D. C. 20525

The three operating sections of PHS are the Bureau of Medical Services, the Bureau of State Services, and the National Institutes of Health.

Within the Bureau of Medical Services, the Division of Hospitals maintains fifteen hospitals and twenty-five outpatient clinics throughout the country. General medical and surgical care is provided in twelve of the fifteen hospitals, while specialized treatment for narcotics addiction is offered in one, for neuropsychiatric disorders in another, and for the treatment and study of leprosy in a third. Ninety-six approved medical internships are available at these hospitals, most of which are qualified teaching institutions. In addition, more than 150 residencies are available in fully accredited programs in a variety of medical specialties.

The Division of Indian Health provides medical care and preventive health services to approximately 340,000 Indians in twenty-three states and 43,000 native Alaskans in isolated villages. Further opportunities within the Bureau of Medical Services include service as a medical officer with the Division of Foreign Quarantine at any of twenty sea and land border ports throughout the world and assignment to the medical programs of other federal agencies, including the Peace Corps.

The Bureau of State Services is the operating bureau for federal-state activities. It has two broad types of programs designed to put tested health methods into application: the identification of health problems and the development of effective methods for their prevention, treatment, and control. The bureau works with state and local health agencies and professional and voluntary groups, assisting in the development of preventive, curative, and restorative services for the general public. Careers for physicians include program specialist, public health administrator, program consultant, and epidemiologist.

The National Institutes of Health is the main research facility of PHS. The research conducted and supported by the institutes accounts for 40 percent of the total medical research expenditure in the United States. The extensive grant program supports research in centers and universities throughout the country in addition to the research carried on at NIH. The five-hundred-bed Clinical Center combined with the institutes offers an extremely wide range of choice and experience to the physician interested in the research aspect of a public health career.

Veterans Administration. Because few women suspect that the Veterans Administration is by far the largest employer of woman physicians in the federal government, a special mention of the agency is in order. The VA operates the nation's, perhaps the world's, largest hospital system, with 166 installations, including hospitals, nursing homes, and other extended-care facilities and outpatient clinics.

Dr. H. M. Engle, chief medical director of the Veterans Administration, believes that the agency is uniquely suitable for the woman physician. "For the physician who does not want to spend full time in practice, who is interested in scheduled assignments, who might have to be mobile because of her husband's assignments . . . with our 166 hospitals in every state of the Union, we can offer opportunities just about everywhere." [18]

Dr. Engle states that, among the medical specialties, the VA's greatest need for personnel is in psychiatry. "Half of our 115,000 hospital beds are in this specialty, and we need all the physician help we can get. In specialties such as anesthesiology and internal medicine, where we also need additional manpower, we have many outpatient clinics where there can be scheduled assignments." [19]

Dr. Engle points out that the VA is unusual in that practically all of its patients are male. Of the twenty-six million war veterans eligible for medical benefits from the VA, the vast majority are male, most in the middle and older age groups. Yet, Dr. Engle reports, in the two decades of his experience he has never been aware of a complaint or concern about woman physicians working with and examining male patients, although other doctors have mentioned such a problem. And so, though reference is sometimes made to the fact that in our culture there is apprehension about woman physicians examining male patients, the experience of the VA shows that it is groundless.[20] This may be attributable in part to the emphasis that the VA has given in recent years to providing equal employment opportunities for women. Institutional approval of such a policy has led to its acceptance by an all-male clientele more quickly than by the general public.

Careers in Public Health at the State and Local Levels. A state's official health agency and the functions it performs vary according to the nature and density of the state's population and its intrinsic urban or rural characteristics. State activities are concerned less with direct medical services than with the consultation, supervision, and training of local health personnel and with planning for improved health services through research, studies, and epidemiologic investigations of health hazards. Physicians with state health departments are apt to be involved in such specialty areas as local health, chronic disease, gerontology, maternal and child health, and mental health. A specialist at this level might be a state commissioner of health who works with many voluntary agencies and

citizens' groups to initiate a statewide program for older persons.
At the local level, the health officer is considered the general practitioner in the community and works in partnership with private physicians to promote the health services of that locality. The woman doctor who becomes a health officer might plan and carry out with her staff such preventive services as community-wide immunization programs, X-ray surveys, glaucoma control activities, and diabetes detection programs. In addition, the public health physician makes decisions about new disease threats that must be overcome and assists in the development of care services for such groups as the chronically ill and the aged. Local public health—the "grass roots of the nation's health"—conducts programs that allow individuals and families to maintain or regain their well-being and usefulness.[21]

Radiology

Radiology is the medical specialty in which X rays and other forms of radiation are used to diagnose and treat diseases and injuries. There are three major areas within the specialty: diagnosis using X rays, radiation therapy for treatment of cancer and other diseases, and the new and rapidly growing field of nuclear medicine. Some radiologists specialize in either diagnosis or therapy; others practice both.[22]

The radiologist "must understand a language of shadows," as one doctor put it.[23] He reads radiographs—what most people call "X-ray pictures." He must know the most minute differences among the various shadows that healthy tissues cast on the film and be able to distinguish them from shadows that may indicate the presence of disease. To do this, the radiologist must first be a competent physician, because only by knowing what is normal and by regarding the patient as a whole person can he interpret the pattern of light and shadow on an X-ray film to reach an accurate diagnosis.

Training to attain such skill is extensive. After medical school and internship, there is a three-year residency that includes training in diagnostic and therapeutic radiology plus the study of radiation physics and radiobiology. Clinical and occasionally basic research is expected. Then, a year after completing the residency, a doctor can take the board-qualifying examination.

Radiologists practice both in hospitals and in private offices. According to a U.S. Public Health Service survey, about half of the radiology is done in hospitals, one-fourth in offices, and one-fourth in public health facilities.[24]

In diagnosis, the radiologist looks for tumors, gallstones, ulcers, broken bones, tuberculosis, heart disease, and many other diseases and malfunctions of the human body. This is accomplished by the study of X-ray films and through fluoroscopy, in which the doctor observes various body organs in motion either directly, on a luminescent screen placed against the patient's body, or indirectly, on a special television set.

In therapy, the radiologist uses high-energy radiation to affect body tissue. This therapy is used primarily against cancer, and employs a high level of radiation in order to kill as many cancer cells as possible while sparing as many healthy cells as possible. Radiation does the most harm to cells that are in the process of dividing; mature cells can recover from short doses of radiation. The treatment is based on the principle that the healthy, mature cells will have time to recover between doses, but that cancer cells, having been hit when it hurts them most, will be unable to grow and, it is hoped, the cancer will then shrivel up and die. X-ray treatment is increasingly being used in combination with surgery and chemical agents.

Nuclear medicine is a new subspecialty of radiology encompassing both diagnosis and treatment. Radioactive substances are used in chemical solutions to diagnose and treat disease. Tiny amounts of radioactive material are injected into the body in a solution, and their course is traced by a counting or scanning device. In some cases, heavier quantities of radioactivity may then be used to treat the condition revealed by the trace amounts. Almost every organ in the body can be scanned, or visualized, through the use of specific radiopharmaceuticals. Because the concentration of the isotope injection differs in healthy and in diseased tissue, the tracings—called "scans"— can depict the distribution of the isotope and thus indicate the condition of the organ.

The demand for personnel in the field of nuclear medicine assures the future of any qualified specialist. Dr. James L. Quinn, vice-president of the central chapter of the Society of Nuclear Medicine, estimates that there is an immediate need for twelve hundred physicians in nuclear medicine and that there are hundreds of opportunities for part-time practitioners in small hospitals. Currently, fewer than five hundred physicians are involved in full-time nuclear medicine. Both the federal government and the profession of radiology are actively working to establish training programs at all levels to increase the number of physicians in nuclear medicine.[25]

Women will readily find a place in the specialty of radiology. The American College of Radiology points out that, although no specific programs have been formulated to assist women in training for the field, "it is worth noting that the coverage of a hospital X-ray department or a multidoctor clinic is frequently arranged on a part-time basis, and this might be particularly suited to a woman physician who is trying to raise a family and practice as well." [26] The board policy occasionally permits part-time residencies, on an individual basis.[27]

Research opportunities in radiology are especially rich and varied, occurring in such fields as radiobiology, radiation physics, radiation chemistry, genetics, circulatory and respiratory physiology, and electronics. Careers in these areas permit activity in teaching, consultation, research, and in institutional appointments—all jobs with manageable hours.

A Ph.D. degree instead of, or in combination with, the M.D. is valuable for some of these careers. Radiology is becoming increasingly dependent on physics and mathematics, and research workers in these fields are contributing heavily to the advances in the specialty.

Radiologic physicists work in research, consultation with physicians, and teaching. They are primarily employed in hospitals, research institutes, government health departments, and industry. They are the only nonphysicians who are examined for certification by a medical specialty board, the American Board of Radiology.[28] These physicists work to develop new and better equipment and techniques, and study methods to measure the amounts of radioactivity in the human body and in foodstuffs.

The radiobiologist (also not necessarily a physician) experiments on animals to study the effects of radiation on various body organs, functions, diseases, and other health problems. These specialists work mostly in large teaching hospitals and medical schools. Medicine in the future will deal more and more with the human body on the cellular level. Doctors will treat not a diseased organ but the few thousand cells immediately affected. Medicine will increase its emphasis on preventive practice. Radiology is important in both of these areas and will have an increasingly larger role in the practice of medicine.

Research

Research opportunities exist in every medical specialty field and in all of the basic sciences. Medical research is the area in which one can most readily apply Thomas Edison's definition of genius as being "1 percent inspiration and 99 percent perspiration." Successful researchers are characterized by the ability to proceed steadily toward their goal through daily work that eliminates the incorrect possibilities, not through sudden flashes of inspiration.

Coupled with the obvious satisfactions of creativity and the occasional moments of discovery is that great advantage for the working wife, regular hours. Research is no more physically demanding, even on a full-time basis, than other professions.

In medical schools and teaching hospitals, research is carried on by members of the faculty, who combine it with their teaching duties. A research worker, who holds an M.D., a Ph.D. in the physical sciences, or both, defines a research problem, sets forth premises and hypotheses, designs the methods of the investigation, and directs a staff of assistants and technicians in carrying out the investigation.

Researchers work in the many institutes and laboratories supported by government agencies. Government grants also support individual projects carried out in the universities and medical schools by eligible investigators.

The extensive research carried out and supported by the National Institutes of Health, of the Public Health Service, is conducted in the areas of: allergy and infectious diseases, arthritis and metabolic diseases, cancer, dental research, heart, mental health, neurological diseases and blindness, child health and human development, and general medical services. As has been stated, the institutes and their broad program of grants to researchers throughout the country account for 40 percent of the total medical research expenditure in the United States.

Private foundations support research on specific diseases, such as cancer, heart disease, asthma, and muscular dystrophy. Pharmaceutical companies have extensive laboratory facilities and support a wide range of research, in addition to awarding grants to individual investigators. Private industry is another area where laboratory research opportunities abound, particularly in the physical sciences such as chemistry and physics.

By its very nature, medicine tends to involve many doctors in research at some stage of their careers. Most of the young woman physicians, and some of the medical students interviewed, expressed interest in a problem that was already beginning to puzzle them and that, in their opinion, called for further investigation. Research, therefore, should not necessarily be viewed as a separate entity, but rather as another aspect of medicine.

A woman may choose to work exclusively in the laboratory if a day-to-day contribution to scientific knowledge is her greatest satisfaction. Another may decide to accept a research position during the child-rearing years so that she can keep in contact with the latest developments in her field of special interest—and do so during acceptable working hours. A third may participate sporadically in research projects as challenges arise. Other women, who dislike the environment of an isolated laboratory because they miss patient contact, find clinical research in an area such as dermatology, ophthalmology, pediatrics, or psychiatry the most suitable for them.

Adjusting to a Dual Career

These career choices are only a few of the many options available to the woman physician. They illustrate the diversity of the field of medicine and the many ways in which a married woman can utilize her M.D. while maintaining her role of wife and mother.

Dr. Margaret Giannini captures the essence of the gradual adjustments that a woman makes throughout life as her needs change:

"[Concern over] the adjustment from career woman to mother presupposes, I think, a problem that does not necessarily exist. The transition from one role to another is not like a tap—turned off or on, hot or cold. It is instinctive—a natural evolution. Of course, I had to work out a system, one that is flexible enough to enable me to *function on all levels*. I enjoy lots of levels and doing what needs to be done."

The ability to handle each task as it presents itself—whether it is delivering an address to a national medical meeting or kissing a bumped knee to make it better—enables the mother-doctor to meet both career and family commitments. The physicians interviewed often mentioned that no one should enter a particular specialty solely because "it is a good career for a woman."

However, some areas are more suitable for the career-marriage combination than others, and a woman should familiarize herself with as many of them as possible before making the final decision on whether or not she can handle both marriage and medicine.

If you are a woman who is planning to be both a doctor and a mother, the following considerations are essential to your success in handling a dual career:

1. Make sure your working hours are predictable. Especially when the children are young, mothers who have institutional appointments or faculty positions, or who are doing laboratory work, find they can devote more time to their families by working regular hours. Many married physicians advocate specialties in which night calls are minimal or nonexistent.

2. Control your intake. Instead of attempting an individual private practice, you can practice in almost any locality in hospitals, in clinics, or in group practice, where emergency calls are shared on a predetermined schedule. Establish the hours you can manage and try not to exceed them.

3. Have competent and reliable household help. As many household duties as possible should be delegated, so that when the mother-physician is at home her time can be devoted to husband and children. She can reserve for herself the domestic duties she most enjoys, such as cooking or sewing, so long as she does not sap the energy she needs to meet the demands of her dual role. Infants and preschool children should have the love and affection of a mother figure in their own mother's absence.

4. Do your postgraduate training on a part-time or extended basis. Seek out the residency and internship programs that permit maternity leave and time off for family needs if childbearing occurs during these years. If you are already in a traditional program and the pressure becomes too great, rather than dropping out of the profession, appeal to your department chairman for a manageable part-time training program.

5. Recognize the diversity possible in your particular field. You do not have to commit yourself to one phase of medical activity for life. A busy mother with young children can take a part-time teaching appointment or combine teaching with research. When the children are in school, she can enter a practice with controlled hours, and turn to full-time practice when the children are grown.

6. Conserve time and energy; don't waste yourself on trivia. Decide what is essential to each role and do it without being distracted by minor details. Learn to say a judicious "no" to activities that are not necessary and that will take away from your ability to handle your career and family commitments.

Notes to Chapter Five

1. *Distribution of Physicians, Hospitals, and Hospital Beds in the U.S., Regional, State, County, Metropolitan Area,* American Medical Association, 1968. P. 13.
2. *Health Manpower Source Book,* Section 18, published by Public Health Service, U.S. Department of Health, Education and Welfare.
3. *Journal of the American Medical Association,* Vol. 198, No. 8, November 21, 1966.
4. *Facts on Prospective and Practicing Women in Medicine,* report prepared for conference on Meeting Medical Manpower Needs: The Fuller Utilization of the Woman Physician. Published by Women's Bureau, U.S. Department of Labor, January, 1968. P. 60, table 10.
5. Personal communication from Albert M. Betcher, M.D., American Society of Anesthesiologists, August 13, 1968.
6. American Board of Anesthesiology requirements for certification.
7. *Dentistry: A Career for Women,* Council on Dental Education of the American Dental Association, 1968.
8. *Ibid.*
9. *Ibid.*
10. Carol Lopate, *Women in Medicine,* Johns Hopkins Press, 1968. P. 134 footnote #1, table 8–2.
11. *The Psychiatrist,* National Association for Mental Health, Inc., New York, 1967.
12. Ruth Anderson Lawrence, M.D., "The Training of Women Physicians," presented at Josiah Macy, Jr., conference on Women for Medicine, Dedham, Mass., October, 1966. P. 6.
13. Lopate, *op. cit.* p. 134.
14. *Ibid.*
15. Lawrence, *op. cit.,* p. 6.
16. Claire F. Ryder, M.D., M.P.H., "Careers in Public Health," *Career Choices for Women in Medicine,* American Medical Women's Association, 1968. Reprinted by permission from *Journal of the American Medical Women's Association.*
17. *Careers: Public Health Service,* Public Health Service, U.S. Department of Health, Education and Welfare, 1964.
18. H. M. Engle, M.D., opening statement at conference on Meeting Medical Manpower Needs: The Fuller Utilization of the Woman Physician, January 12–13, 1968, Washington, D.C. Sponsored by American Medical Women's Association, President's Study Group on Careers for Women, Women's Bureau of U.S. Department of Labor. Report published by American Medical Women's Association, 1968. Pp. 47–48. Reprinted by permission.
19. *Ibid.*
20. *Ibid.*
21. Claire F. Ryder, M.D., M.P.H. "Careers in Public Health" *Career Choices for Women in Medicine,* Journal of American Medical Women's Association. 1968. Special thanks are offered to the American Medical Women's Association and to Claire F. Ryder, M.D., M.P.H., whose article served as the source for material in the preceding write-up on the field of public health. Reprinted by permission.
22. *Careers in Radiology,* American College of Radiology, Chicago, 1968.
23. *Radiology and Health,* E. I. du Pont de Nemours & Company, with American College of Radiology, 1968.
24. *Ibid.*

25. *Your Radiologist,* American College of Radiology, Chicago, 1968. P. 17.
26. Personal communication from Otha W. Linton, American College of Radiology, August 26, 1968.
27. Lopate, *op. cit.,* p. 134.
28. *Careers in Radiology.*

Chapter Six

HOW NOT TO DO IT
—AND SUCCEED!

If you read all the foregoing advice, distill it into a few maxims, and then do just the opposite, you will have proof that each individual must still chart her own course according to her peculiar needs.

How to succeed without really trying the traditional ways is illustrated by the career of Dr. Mabel K. Gibby. A clinical counseling psychologist at the Veterans Administration Hospital in Miami, Florida, she carries a case load of psychological testing, counseling, and evaluation of severely disturbed patients and also performs duties in vocational rehabilitation. In the latter area, veterans with service-connected nervous disorders are retrained and the handicapped are assisted with vocational goals and then placed in suitable jobs—with the help of this vivacious little blonde mother.

"I am most enthusiastic about a career such as mine for women, because, unlike the physician, I have no night calls. This is a forty-hour-work-week, desk-type job. Yet psychology lets me do a professional kind of activity without taking away from my family."

Clinical psychologists practice psychotherapy and in a hospital usually have charge of diagnostic testing. They often do research to evaluate old procedures and develop new ones. This is not the same task as that of the psychiatrist, a physician who has completed medical training and then specialized in psychiatry.

Dr. Gibby, who started out to be a missionary, took an M.A. in religious education and met her future husband while she was working with a group of young adults. They married while he was in college, she worked while he completed medical school, and then she switched her field to educational guidance and counseling, necessitating a great deal more study. The impossible took her only two years: completion of both another master's degree and a doctorate, and the discovery that an academic gown makes a fine maternity outfit.

"By the time I was twenty-six, I had my first baby, three years of full-time experience in education and social work, and three graduate degrees."

Dr. Gibby had severed all financial ties with her family at the age of nineteen, upon earning her B.A., and used scholarship assistance for all her graduate tuition. She worked in settlement houses and put in many extra hours of field social work at a low hourly rate to earn money for her living expenses.

For young women planning careers in the area of mental health, psychology, and social work, things are far different now. Tax-free stipends are readily available to ambitious students and have increased every year—"they are handed out almost on a silver platter to qualified applicants." Often the hourly rates work out to more than the pay of some full-time departmental staff members.

Dr. Gibby's advice to young girls planning to enter the medical profession is to break out of the traditional educational format, to accelerate their studies at the lower levels while they are young.

"I would encourage girls to use shortcuts in getting through school. I know this is not a popular theory with educators, but it works, particularly with the above-average student. Get it over with in your teens and get out!"

If possible, and if your school permits such a program, finish high school in three years. If your state laws forbid this, investigate the possibility of taking college-level subjects during the summer and later transferring the credits to a college that will accept them. Caution: You must be sure to check with the college of your choice if you plan to pursue such a program, as the degree-granting institution has the final say on acceptance of all college-level credits. However, this program does exist in many areas and is very workable for the student who does not want to while away her senior year in home ec.

In college, you can take courses all year long and finish in three years if you are aiming at medical school or the Ph.D. This can be accomplished through attendance at summer school or, in the trimester system, through year-round enrollment. With the growing need in all professions for persons with graduate degrees, this program is no longer revolutionary and many students are completing it successfully.

Dr. Gibby accelerated her graduate studies, but she points out that the course work at that level is much more demanding, whereas lower-level work can often be speeded up without a great deal of effort. The earlier the decision to enter medicine is made, the more time you can save in your preparation.

"If you push through your undergraduate years on the same basis as I did when I finally decided on my career, you can gain a year or even two years of your life. From a practical standpoint— for women—the problems and difficulties are minimal compared with what you endure if you marry and try to finish your education after the children come."

The Gibbys followed the sun to Florida (from St. Louis, Missouri). Her husband, John, began praticing pediatrics, and Mabel Gibby applied for a public school counseling job.

"There was a county rule that they could not hire pregnant women. The official attitude was that this condition embarrassed the children."

Since she was again in an "embarrassing condition," Dr. Gibby accepted an appointment with the Veterans Administration, which doesn't object to expectant mothers, and began her career of ten richly rewarding years as a clinical psychologist. The Gibbys now have seven children.

"I feel that having a job has given *me* a therapeutic experience, too. I could not have so many children if I were home scrubbing floors all day. I would be too tired to have any fun with them."

Mabel Gibby relies on a baby-sitter to care for the younger children while she is out of the house. Upon returning home, she takes over, doing her own cooking, ironing, and sewing. She makes many of her youngsters' clothes, and as a hobby restores fine old tapestries.

Conflicts between woman's role in the home and a demanding professional career?

"No matter how solid the family is, there are always conflicts of interest in the activities of various members," Dr. Gibby says. "Women have to rid themselves of the built-in guilt feelings they have when they leave the home for the business or professional world."

A mother should not relate to her job every difficulty she has with her children. You are not really rejected every time your teenager cries, "You don't understand me"—whether you are a doctor, a secretary, or a housewife.

One of the things most women tend to overlook is that we all have ambivalent feelings toward many things, Dr. Gibby feels. Recognition of this, and knowing that conflicts and crises will come and will inevitably be reflected in the behavior of other members of the family unit, can help you to remain tolerant.

"I remember seeing a cartoon depicting a harassed mother standing amid chaos in her kitchen, crying to her husband, 'I gave him away.' There are times when we all want to 'give them away' and, conversely, times when they don't need you, either—and show it. So long as a mother does not let her job interfere with the things her children feel are really important, she is on safe ground."

The combining of marriage and a profession really demands the ability to divide your time between both without adversely affecting either.

"It gets to the point where your life becomes a little bit dichotomized. Since both my husband and I work with people all day and come into the home only to be surrounded by children, when we are alone we do something that is quiet or pursue individual creative activities. Our spare time is spent just being with each other. There is too much stress being put on togetherness today. We do not belong to clubs or organizations or go to parties."

Weekends at the Gibby home sound like a description of Camp Runamuck with cultural overtones. The Gibby children may entertain as many as six or seven friends who stay overnight and are overwhelmingly present for all meals. Mabel Gibby wants her home to be a place where guests, particularly young friends, can arrive at mealtime and she only needs to put on another plate.

"We are the only people in town with a wall-to-wall table. Our huge twelve-foot dining room table is full to capacity at most meals. I think this dining table, more than anything, symbolizes our family life."

Recognition of Dr. Gibby's achievements has been nationwide. She was named Top Professional Rehabilitation Worker in the United States and has received county and state honors. Her current research project concerns the correlation of records of handicapped job applicants and suitable employment. When it is completed, the data will first be used by the Cape Kennedy Space Center in Florida and then expanded into a statewide project.

Dr. Gibby is a realist. She knows she must stay in her present locality, where her husband's practice is established. She cannot apply for a higher-level job in her profession that would take her away from the Miami hospital.

"I put these limits on myself. A woman *must* put limits on her success if she wants a family. I feel we women are lucky. We can 'have our cake and eat it, too.' With the large family I always wanted, a big, happy home, and a job I like, I feel I am as successful as I wanted to be when I started out to become a doctor."

PART II

THE MEDICAL PROFESSION

Chapter Seven

ADMISSION REQUIREMENTS OF MEDICAL SCHOOLS

"Each medical school hopes that each student admitted will successfully complete the four years of study required for his M.D. degree. If a student fails or withdraws from a class, he cannot be replaced. The end result is that one less physician will be graduated." [1]

With two applicants for every available seat in medical school, admissions committees are careful to select only those students who show the greatest promise, both of academic success and of motivation to complete their education and serve the profession throughout their lifetime.

Know What You Are Looking For in a Medical School

Medical schools vary considerably, not in the basic curriculum but in philosophy of education, emphasis given various areas of study, size of student body, student-faculty ratio, and facilities for clinical study and research. The geographical location of a particular school can be an asset to the career you intend to pursue. If the school is located in a large metropolitan center, you will observe and treat in its clinics a wide variety of diseases from the surrounding urban neighborhoods; a rural location will provide a different range of health problems.

Medical schools also vary in the types of postgraduate study offered and in the careers their graduates enter. A woman who was graduated from a medical college in the Northeast pointed out that she had entered academic medicine because her school emphasized the importance of this career and provided ample opportunity to explore and train for it.

Medical colleges are not equal in the talent they attract; not all receive applications from a sufficient number of top students. Many lesser-known schools in the South and West do not have to reject hundreds of applicants when filling their entering classes, as do the well-known schools in the Northeast.

A study by Davis G. Johnson, Ph.D., on medical school applicants, published in the *Journal of the American Medical Association,* covered several of these points; it is summarized as follows:

"The intellectual caliber of applicants as measured by the MCAT [Medical College Admission Test] remains at a high level. Schools in the South have the lowest number of applicants, with the highest number being concentrated in the Northeast. Women are accepted in an almost identical rate to male applicants, proportionate to the number of applications submitted." [2]

All medical schools admit women, and the Woman's Medical College of Pennsylvania, as its name suggests, admits women only. This does not mean, however, that all the schools are equal in their attitude or policies toward accepting women. Prejudice often operates subtly, and it would be wise to familiarize yourself with those schools where the number of women accepted is limited by either policy or attitude.

An example of prejudicial attitude is the variance in the admission requirements for applicants to particular schools. One school has just introduced a new mathematics requirement for entrance because the administration feels that "one cannot be a respectable scientist, cannot do a good job in any field in the life sciences, without a mathematical and physical base."

In general, the talents of women do not fall into the physical and mathematical sciences. As the dean of admissions at this school states: "The inclinations of women are not on this track. The average score on the MCAT in the math portion of the test is lower than for the corresponding male." To date, this school has been liberal in its acceptance of woman students, but the new requirement will very likely operate against them in the future.

Women should be aware that extreme attitudes do exist at some colleges. Many admissions committees hold the view that, since there are sufficient numbers of qualified men who will make a greater quantitative return to the profession, women should not even be considered. One dean stated flatly that "we have no business taking women into medical school at all"—and he is conducting an active campaign against them by corresponding with his friends on admissions committees throughout the country in an attempt to win them to his view.

Many schools evaluate candidates without regard to sex, and the fact that women are so much in the minority reflects the fact that a much smaller number of women than of men apply to medical school. Dean Gerald A. Green of the University of Southern California (which has a high percentage of woman medical students) explains the situation:

"The fact that racial and ethnic minorities are underrepresented [in medical school classes] throughout the nation I would attribute to the fact that they are underrepresented in the applicant pool. Although . . . this applies to women to a lesser degree, a look at our statistics over the past several years indicates that the percentage of women now entering USC exceeds the percentage of women in the applicant pool. Nevertheless, this has not been the result of conscious favorable bias toward women.

"According to a recent issue of *Medical World News,* USC has a larger percentage of women in its student body than any other medical school except Woman's Medical College. . . . No specific attempt is being made to increase the number of women in our student body—it just works out that way.

"Obviously, more qualified women are applying to our school all the time, and these increased numbers in the applicant pool reflect themselves in the [Admissions] Committee's resultant decisions. . . .

"The numbers of women in the entering classes will increase as women come to think of medicine as a legitimate career field and one to which they can reasonably aspire." [3]

When selecting her premedical college, a girl should keep in mind that medical school admissions committees will evaluate the strength of the science department and the reputation of its faculty. Admissions committees tend to be skeptical about "A" grades in chemistry from colleges that emphasize the humanities at the expense of high-quality science instruction. A girl with a "B" average from a college with a topflight science curriculum will have an advantage over a girl with an "A" average from a college whose science departments are less highly rated. This does not mean that a girl cannot take a nonscientific major; she can, as long as she completes all the required science courses in a topflight department. Weak science and math preparation will show up in her MCAT scores.

It is imperative for every potential medical school applicant to secure a personal copy of *Medical School Admission Requirements* for the purpose of evaluating all the schools. This book provides an up-to-date and official source of information on premedical preparation and admission to medical school. In addition to informative chapters on the medical school admission process, the publication lists every accredited medical school in the United States and Canada, with individual admission requirements and a valuable profile of each school with respect to its educational philosophy, selection criteria, special study and training programs, and financial information. The General Information section of the individual school's description enables the prospective applicant to assess her chances for acceptance and determine whether or not the school offers her desired course of study.

The book is issued each year in late summer and can be obtained for four dollars per copy from:

> Association of American Medical Colleges
> 2530 Ridge Avenue
> Evanston, Illinois 60201

Medical School Admission Requirements also contains many valuable tables that will clarify the admission policies of each school. One table, entitled "Medical School Preferences with Respect to Sex, Race, Residence, and Age of Applicants," sets forth some of the factors that may work against an applicant at one school but make her welcome at another.

One example is age. The AAMC states: "Age can be a distinctly limiting factor in gaining admission to medical school—so much so that the older premedical student should consider very carefully before continuing in his educational preparation for medicine . . . stated age limits range from ages 16 to 35 years. The median preferred age range . . . is 20 to 26 years." [4] Woman's Medical College keeps an open mind regarding age, and will accept qualified woman applicants who are older than the average if they wish to pursue careers in medicine after raising their children.

Race is not a factor in screening applicants, but two medical schools, Howard and Meharry, admit mostly Negroes. Howard's policy states that "Howard is open to all races but favors the admission of Negroes because of restricted opportunities for Negroes elsewhere." [5] As premedical educational opportunities for Negro students increase, more of them are finding their way into the applicant pool at all schools, and this whole situation is undergoing change.

Residency Requirements
Some of the most inflexible limitations on acceptance are those pertaining to residence. State-supported medical schools are required by law to give preference to residents of their states, either by a definite quota system or by informal preference combined with acceptance of some out-of-state students. Residents usually pay much lower tuition in tax-supported schools. The individual schools' restrictions and advantages pertaining to residency requirements are itemized in the AAMC publication.

Students from western states that have no medical schools may apply for assistance in attending schools that participate in the student exchange program of the Western Interstate Commission for Higher Education. The state in which the eligible student resides makes a payment to the desired medical school on his behalf. Applications must be filed with the student's state of residence. Further information can be obtained by writing to the commission at: University East Campus, 30th Street, Boulder, Colorado 80302.

The AAMC advises that such restrictions should not deter a student from submitting applications to schools outside his home state. Just keep in mind that such restrictions exist, familiarize yourself with the policies of different schools, and consider the advantages of a change of environment if a particular school seems to suit your interests and abilities. The AAMC states:

"The medical schools are considered to be a national resource and the successful graduate of any can establish private practice in practically any state or region of the United States without difficulty. Indeed, a deliberate change of geographic environment . . . may be quite useful in gaining breadth of culture and education." [6]

How Medical Schools Evaluate Their Applicants
Students are evaluated on the basis of four major factors:

    1. premedical credits as reflected in the candidate's college transcript;

2. the MCAT score;
3. the application form, including a confidential evaluation from the candidate's college (particularly from his premedical adviser) of his undergraduate work, plus written references regarding personal integrity and academic ability;
4. the personal interview.

Premedical Credits. Most medical schools require a minimum of three years of undergraduate college work. Ten schools require a degree, and many more recommend it. It is possible at almost two-thirds of the schools to complete degree requirements after enrollment in medical school. The Association of American Medical Colleges states that college grades are perhaps the most important single indicator of medical school performance. When evaluating undergraduate grades, admissions committees take into consideration the institution the applicant attended. In some cases, "C" students are accepted if they have attended strong colleges with strict grading policies in the sciences. The majority of medical schools, however, prefer to consider only students with grade averages no lower than "B minus" or the equivalent.[7]

Admissions committees take into consideration the type of course load the student carried and the college's academic standards. Other factors weighed are the number of honors courses taken and whether the student worked part-time while in college.

It is well for the premedical student to use caution in the amount of time he spends on extracurricular activities or part-time work during his undergraduate years. Since premedical grades are important, the student should not burden himself to the point that he cannot keep his grade average at a level consistent with his ability.

Advanced Placement. "Advanced placement is the allowance of college credit for college-level courses taken in high school and attested by scores on the Advanced Placement Examinations of the College Entrance Examination Board or on similar examinations administered directly by the college." [8]

It is the responsibility of the individual student to see that these credits are in order and are recorded on his college transcript. The student should also make sure that his premedical adviser informs the colleges to which he has applied of his participation in an advanced placement program.

The Association of American Medical Colleges has published

the following recommendations regarding advanced placement credits:

> ". . . *undergraduate colleges* should be encouraged to: (a) clearly indicate on the official college transcript how much credit has been allowed for each of such courses toward the bachelor's degree, and (b) advise such premedical students to pursue advanced courses in biology, chemistry, or physics in college if they met the minimum science requirements while in high school.
>
> "That *medical schools* should be encouraged to: (a) accept advanced placement credits for admission to medical school if the credits are clearly indicated on the undergraduate college transcript as having been accepted by the college toward fulfillment of requirements for the bachelor's degree, and (b) publicize the above in appropriate medical school admissions publications.
>
> "That *State Licensing Boards* should be encouraged to: (a) accept advanced placement credits as prerequisites for medical licensure if they are clearly designated on the undergraduate college transcript, and if they have been accepted by an accredited medical school as meeting its admission requirements, and (b) seek the inclusion of such a policy statement in their licensure regulations." [9]

The Medical College Admission Test (MCAT). All medical schools in the United States either require or strongly recommend that all students planning to apply for admission take the Medical College Admission Test. The test is given twice a year, in the spring (April or May) and in the fall (October). Most schools prefer that the test be taken in the spring (in the student's junior year of undergraduate study).

Careful preparation for this examination is essential. You should complete as many of the required science courses as possible before taking the test. The Association of American Medical Colleges states that "the MCAT provides admissions committees with nationally standardized measures of both scholastic ability and achievement. This enables a medical school to compare applicants, even though they may have widely differing personal and academic backgrounds. MCAT scores provide . . . important information on academic capabilities for the study of medicine and permit more thorough interpretation of the college academic record." [10]

Several books are available to help students prepare for the MCAT, including *How to Pass Medical College Admission Test,* published by Cowles Book Company, Inc., LOOK Building, 488 Madison Avenue, New York, New York 10022. This publication is available at campus and other book stores, or directly from the publisher, at $3.95 per copy.

It is the responsibility of the student to make his own arrangements for taking the test. An announcement booklet is prepared annually by the Psychological Corporation, which administers the test, that contains an application blank, information concerning test dates, deadlines for application, testing locations, and sample questions. The booklet is available in the offices of many college premedical advisers, or it may be obtained by writing to:

> Medical College Admission Test
> The Psychological Corporation
> 304 East 45th Street
> New York, New York 10017

Complete the application blank and submit it with the twenty-dollar examination fee, which entitles each candidate to have his test score sent to six medical schools. If additional scores are required, the student may request them at one dollar each. One report is transmitted to the examinee at no additional charge, so that the student may submit it to his premedical adviser.

The Application. "The application form itself is one of the most important sources of information that admissions committees utilize in considering applicants. It should be filled out completely and accurately, and neatness and legibility of entries are important." [11]

The American Medical Association advises students to submit applications to several schools, to better their chances for acceptance. The current national average of applications per candidate is four.[12] Select with care the schools to which you apply, evaluating their programs and comparing them with your qualifications. Plan your strategy carefully to include one or two schools that are not among the prestige schools, with their overabundance of highly qualified candidates. Consider a variety of geographical areas. Check with your premedical adviser for further suggestions and assistance.

Application forms (or kits that contain a number of forms) vary from school to school, but all require information on the candidate's personal history and education. They usually request all or some of the following data: scholastic honors, extracurricular activities, financial information, family history, and health history. Schools receiving state tax funds require an affidavit of residence from the student and from one or two other persons (not relatives). Often a brief composition (about 250 words) is requested in which the student is asked to describe his reasons for wanting to become a physician. A photograph is usually required; pay attention to the size and pose specified.

In addition, it is the responsibility of the applicant to see that his college transcript is forwarded to each medical school to which he applies. An evaluation form may be attached to the application; this form must be filled out by the premedical adviser at the undergraduate college. Instead of the evaluation, or in addition to it, the applicant usually is required to solicit letters of recommendation from two or three science faculty members. Read carefully the specifications for letters of evaluation, as they vary from school to school. Notify each professor whose name you are submitting as a reference, and do *not* submit additional recommendations if they are not requested by the medical school.

The confidential evaluation of the student's qualifications is sent by the premedical adviser directly to the medical school. Both academic and personal factors are considered, usually rated on a scale ranging from "superior" through "poor," with space for special comments. Some of the criteria on which you will be rated are: judgment or common sense, scholastic ability, integrity, ability to get along with people, stability, consistency of effort, neatness, speech, poise, courtesy, initiative, leadership, tact, originality, efficient use of time, willingness to cooperate, and as many other traits as admissions committees have the time or the creativity to think of. A list of your weaknesses may also be requested.

Plan to submit your applications and all the required supporting data approximately one year before the date you expect to enter medical school. Application and acceptance timetables for individual medical schools are given in the AAMC admission requirements book, as is a summary of the policies of the various schools with regard to dates of application. The AAMC warns that the majority of schools will not initiate consideration of an application later than December, and you should plan to apply well before then. Be sure to include the required fee (usually ten dollars) with each application submitted; this is *not* refundable.

The Personal Interview. The medical school usually takes the initiative in requesting an applicant to come to the campus for a personal interview. If the student is expected to request the interview, the application form will specify the procedure to follow. When time and personal finances do not permit a visit to a distant medical school, sometimes arrangements can be made for a local physician—usually an alumnus of that school—to conduct the interview. In such special situations, the arrangements should be handled promptly by correspondence.

The interview serves a constructive purpose for the medical school and for the applicant, and it should not be regarded as an ordeal. You are going to look the school over at the same time as the school is considering you. During the interview, both you and the admissions committee will have an opportunity to clarify the information regarding your background and your application, and you will be able to elaborate on any complicated details in the material you submitted. You should ask pertinent questions about anything concerning the school, its curriculum, philosophy, or student body that is not clear to you. Do not, however, dominate the interview or ask trivial questions. Let the admissions officer guide the interview. Answer his questions directly and pleasantly. Demonstrate confidence in your capabilities without being arrogant; show enthusiasm without being effusive. If you sincerely believe that the medical school you are visiting is the right one for you, and that you will be a valuable member of the medical profession, your interest and capabilities will not escape the interviewer.

Some or all of the following topics will come up during the interview, and the applicant should be ready with thoughtful, well-prepared answers. The woman applicant in particular may find that she is expected to demonstrate a higher degree of motivation and dedication than the male applicant, who will be pursuing his career for a lifetime role as the breadwinner.

You probably will be confronted with statistics on dropout rates and nonpractice rates of woman physicians. Although the national rates are higher for women than men,[13] the University of Miami (Florida) did an independent study on medical school dropouts there and discovered no difference between women and men: females at the University of Miami did not have any higher dropout rate than males.

As for the committee's questions about dropping out of practice once your medical education is completed—and this is a particularly sensitive point to tax-supported schools—be ready to show in a general way how you plan to handle the two careers of physician and mother. Do not deny that you want children, or state that you will not marry until your training is completed. Such thinking is not considered normal for women and would reflect less favorably on you than a positive and workable plan to combine both roles.

The more idealistic schools may actually favor a woman's motives for entering medicine, believing that it is her sincere interest in the profession and her desire to serve humanity that have attracted her to the field, not just the prospect of a lucrative and prestigious career.

The following are examples of questions of a general nature that you may have to answer: How do you organize your time; your studies? How do you plan to manage your money; your living arrangements? Why did you select medicine as a career? How do you plan to use your education after graduation? What are your outside interests?

From your attitude and answers, the interviewer will try to determine if you can get along with people. He will look for "evidence of good interpersonal relationships," as one dean put it. Would you be able to work well with others, or at least not be an aggravation in work situations?

One of the most important factors evaluated during the personal interview is motivation. This ambiguous term crops up with emphasis and regularity in descriptions of what medical schools seek in their applicants. The word is given various interpretations in different schools.

As applied to the female medical school applicant, motivation generally means the strength of her determination to stay in the profession if she is accepted. Whether openly or by implication, most admissions committees demand this kind of motivation more from female candidates than from male, because of the obvious attraction for women of marriage and motherhood. It is assumed that the men will stay in the profession because their traditional role is to support the family. Women who compete for the limited seats in medical schools are expected to demonstrate their willingness to stick with the career once they are educated, and to back up this dedication with some solid solutions to the career-marriage conflict.

One dean defined motivation as sincerity, or dedication of purpose, and supplied the following illustration of the kind of applicant he tries to avoid:

"I know of a medical school where a girl who was in her senior year did not apply for internship at the proper time. A staff member stopped her in the hall between classes and asked her why she had failed to do so. The girl told him, 'I'm going to get my M.D. on the morning of graduation, and then I'm getting married in the afternoon—and that's that!' She ruined the chances for acceptance of women at that school for a good many years, until the case was forgotten." Obviously, it is still not forgotten, or the story never would have been told.

In addition to the applicant's strong desire to stay in the profession and serve, different schools seek different types of students and favor a variety of motives for entering medicine. Factors such as the size of the school, the type of research emphasized, the educational philosophy, and the special programs it has developed influence the selection of students. At the same time, each school tries to include a variety of personality types in every entering class.

To gain the widest possible sample of what the medical schools are looking for, lengthy interviews were conducted in different parts of the country, augmented by correspondence and questionnaires. Many deans of admissions and college administrators responded with lengthy written and verbal opinions, expressions of policy (particularly toward women), projected plans for the makeup of future entering classes, and their definitions of motivation. Some of their most cogent and representative opinions follow:

"We prefer students who have a great deal of interest in community medicine. We look for this motive. We would like to see more being done for the people in the ghettoes; this arises in a school affiliated with a large metropolitan hospital. We are also interested in students motivated to give service abroad, in the underdeveloped countries. I find the young people are often far ahead of the faculty in their conception of role, of service; these motives are coming up more frequently now.

"We also look for a willingness to work in rural areas; the idea of taking an assignment in rural communities never occurs to most young men. Linked to the idea of more doctors is a more appropriate distribution of doctors. You can't tell people where they can work; you can't compel people to do this. But you can look for young people with civic conscience. I feel this new generation has more civic conscience than those who came before.

"I am against indicating a proportion of women students to men, or a certain percentage of Negroes, etc. I do not believe in admitting percentages of any given minority just because they are part of that minority. New York Medical College makes no distinction between the sexes. Here, an older woman can get in if she has the background and motivation. The motivation comes through at the interview."—Dr. David Denker, *President, New York Medical College.*

The colleges are aware that some of the idealism and motivation can become corrupted as the student progresses through his education and is exposed to more facets of the profession.

"The ideas of the entrepreneur filter down to the freshmen and sophomores and influence their decision on their specialty."—Dr. Denker.

"Once in an interview when I was telling an applicant that the medical profession is usually conservative, the student said, 'This is your fault—the fault of the attitudes of admissions committees nationwide. Why don't they admit more liberal-minded students?'

"I replied that I didn't think this was true—that only conservative types were selected for medical school. I think our admissions committee is favorably disposed toward liberal applicants. Only those individuals who are highly individualistic are attracted to the profession in the first place.

"Medical students almost invariably lose their idealism. Their attitudes undergo a change between the time they enter medical school and the time they enter practice. I think this is inevitable. One cannot be constantly exposed to human suffering without becoming somewhat hardened to it."—Dr. George Lewis, *Associate Dean, University of Miami School of Medicine.*

"In addition to academic proficiency, we are greatly concerned with such difficult-to-measure qualities in our applicants as desire to serve, desire to innovate, attitude of flexibility about health care delivery. . . . It is not at all unusual for us to reject applicants with high academic qualifications if they do not display these other qualities. We attempt to adduce data on these qualities by extensive interviews with applicants."—Gerald Allen Green, *Ph.D., Associate Dean for Admissions, University of Southern California.*

"We would hope that the physician will always think in terms of the patient. We look for motivation toward patient-oriented teaching, research, or service."—Dean of Admissions, *University of Kansas School of Medicine.*

"Ideally, we need individuals who are honest, who wish to contribute to the welfare of others, who maintain their intellectual curiosity, and who use good judgment.

"Motivation is too obscure a term to have any real meaning. The external evidence is 'drive' and willingness to work. The internal dynamics can be for 'good' or 'bad' reasons."—Associate Dean, *Bowman Gray School of Medicine, Wake Forest College, North Carolina.*

"The goal of all medical schools is to train students who will contribute to the profession in one way or another, and the female physician will find ready acceptance of her talents within the field of medicine, provided she remains motivated to contribute, whether married or single. Medicine has many different opportunities to choose from, including part-time professional service with institutions and organizations.

"I look forward to more good [female] applicants, because the woman medical students always are a delight to have in class. They're excellent students, and they keep the males, students and faculty alike, on their toes for a variety of reasons which need no discussion. . . ."—John H. Wulsin, M.D., *Admissions Committee, University of Cincinnati College of Medicine.*[14]

A few medical educators are beginning to question the strong emphasis being placed on dedication to the profession, and the "double helping" expected of women. Do we overwarn our ambitious, strongly motivated girls about the occupational perils ahead in medicine, engineering, and the other professions? The irregular hours and considerable demands of a nursing career are accepted as being suitable for women, yet when it comes to the woman doctor we tend to emphasize the difficulty of scheduling and work hours.

Dr. Mary I. Bunting, president of Radcliffe College, tells of a conference she participated in several years ago for women in science:

"They had gathered a splendid group of college students in the sciences and talked to them for hours on the importance of commitment. When I had lunch with the students afterward, I discovered that the immediate effect had been to discourage them. They didn't consider themselves *that* motivated. I realized that bright young men would not be subjected to any such hurdle." [15]

Sincerity is one of the most important qualities, plus a genuine interest in medicine. But you are not expected to feel a saintly renunciation of things worldly in favor of a transcending interest in things medical.

"The qualifications for being a doctor are almost the same whether one is a man or a woman. It requires a certain degree of intelligence. It requires also dedication, a sense of responsibility, and an enjoyment of hard work," Dr. Dorothy V. Whipple told the conference on the Fuller Utilization of the Woman Physician.[16]

The candidate should be able to project these qualities in human, not superhuman, quantities. It is the opinion of Dr. Whipple that all these qualifications are, on the average, a little more evident in the girls who complete their medical training.

"One finds that some men whose talents might be considered mediocre do succeed in medicine, but mediocre women either do not start on a medical career or are discouraged and drop out along the way. As a result, there are very few mediocre woman doctors." [17]

The refusal of some male faculty and admission committee members to recognize in what ways girl students are different from boys causes erroneous attitudes. In the screening of medical school applicants, emphasis often is placed on equality rather than on comparability; there is a refusal to look at significant differences, whether innate or acquired. "Our medical school faculties often assume that a woman should perform exactly the same as a man. I believe this is probably one factor that has caused some of the problems women experience in attempting to complete their medical education," says Dr. Lee Powers, associate director of the Association of American Medical Colleges.[18]

Women should be aware of the mixed bag of attitudes and emotions prevalent in medical schools today so that they can best cope with the questions that will come their way during the admission process. This background of information will help them to evaluate their own motives and potential, and provide guidelines for self-expression.

Acceptance

A student should not hold more than one acceptance to a medical school at any one time. Because most students submit multiple applications, and because competition for the limited number of seats is considerable, most schools require that a student make a substantial deposit (usually fifty dollars) upon acceptance of an offer of admission. This deposit is applied to the first year's tuition. It is usually refundable until January 15 of the year preceding the beginning of his first year. Cancellation of acceptance after that date (or any other date specified by the individual school) results in forfeiture of the fee. If a student receives acceptances from two or more schools, he should make his choice promptly and notify the other schools of his decision to withdraw.

Notes to Chapter Seven

1. *Horizons Unlimited,* American Medical Association, 1968. P. 23.
2. *Journal of the American Medical Association,* Vol. 198, No. 8, November 21, 1966. Figures and comparisons also made from same study published in 1965: Davis G. Johnson, Ph.D., "The Study of Applicants, 1964–1965," *Journal of Medical Education,* Vol. 40, November, 1965.
3. Personal communication from Gerald A. Green, Ph.D., Associate Dean for Admissions, University of Southern California School of Medicine, July 23, 1968.
4. *Medical School Admission Requirements,* 1968–1969, Association of American Medical Colleges. Pp. 9–12, table 2.1. Reprinted by permission.
5. *Ibid.*
6. *Ibid.*
7. *Horizons Unlimited.* Pp. 24, 25.
8. *Medical School Admission Requirements,* 1968–1969. P. 19, table 3.1. Reprinted by permission.
9. *Ibid.*
10. *Op. cit.* P. 21.
11. *Op. cit.* P. 23.
12. *Horizons Unlimited.* Pp. 24, 25.
13. *Datagrams,* Association of American Medical Colleges, Vol. 7, No. 8, February, 1966.
14. John H. Wulsin, M.D., "Admission of Women to Medical School," *Journal of the American Medical Women's Association,* Vol. 21, No. 8, August, 1966. Pp. 674–676.
15. "The College Years," Mary I. Bunting, Ph.D., from report of conference on Meeting Medical Manpower Needs: The Fuller Utilization of the Woman Physician, January 12–13, 1968, Washington D.C. Sponsored by American Medical Women's Association, President's Study Group on Careers for Women, Women's Bureau of U.S. Department of Labor. Published by American Medical Women's Association, 1968. Pp. 23–26. Reprinted by permission.
16. Dorothy V. Whipple, M.D., "Practice and Family Life," *op. cit.* Pp. 33–34.
17. *Ibid.*
18. Lee Powers, M.D., "Remarks," *op. cit.* Pp. 55–57.

Chapter Eight

U.S. AND AFFILIATED
MEDICAL SCHOOLS

Schools of medicine in the United States are listed below, alphabetically by state, since residency is often a factor when considering applicants. Schools of medicine in Puerto Rico, and the Philippines, and at the American University in Lebanon, are included at the end of the listing; these are affiliated with the Association of American Medical Colleges, as are the Canadian schools that follow in a separate list. Graduates of these schools are considered for licensing in the United States on the same basis as graduates of American medical schools. The warnings regarding foreign medical schools set forth in Chapter 11 do not apply to these affiliated schools.[1]

United States Schools
Alabama
  Medical College of Alabama
Arizona
  University of Arizona College of Medicine
Arkansas
  University of Arkansas School of Medicine
California
  University of California, Davis, School of Medicine
  University of California, Irvine, California College of Medicine
  University of California at Los Angeles (UCLA) School of
    Medicine

University of California at San Diego School of Medicine
University of California School of Medicine, San Francisco
Loma Linda University School of Medicine
University of Southern California School of Medicine
Stanford University School of Medicine
Colorado
University of Colorado School of Medicine
Connecticut
University of Connecticut School of Medicine
Yale University School of Medicine
District of Columbia
Georgetown University School of Medicine
George Washington University School of Medicine
Howard University College of Medicine
Florida
University of Florida College of Medicine
University of Miami School of Medicine
University of South Florida (Tampa) Colleges of Medicine &
Nursing
Georgia
Emory University School of Medicine
Medical College of Georgia
Hawaii
University of Hawaii School of Medicine
Illinois
Chicago Medical School
University of Chicago School of Medicine
University of Illinois College of Medicine
Northwestern University Medical School
Stritch School of Medicine, Loyola University
Indiana
Indiana University School of Medicine
Iowa
University of Iowa College of Medicine
Kansas
University of Kansas School of Medicine
Kentucky
University of Kentucky College of Medicine
University of Louisville School of Medicine
Louisiana
Louisiana State University School of Medicine

Louisiana State University Medical Center, Shreveport School
   of Medicine
Tulane University School of Medicine
Maryland
   Johns Hopkins University School of Medicine
   University of Maryland School of Medicine
Massachusetts
   Boston University School of Medicine
   Harvard Medical School
   University of Massachusetts School of Medicine
   Tufts University School of Medicine
Michigan
   University of Michigan Medical School
   Michigan State University College of Human Medicine
   Wayne State University School of Medicine
Minnesota
   University of Minnesota Medical School
Mississippi
   University of Mississippi School of Medicine
Missouri
   University of Missouri School of Medicine
   St. Louis University School of Medicine
   Washington University School of Medicine
Nebraska
   Creighton University School of Medicine
   University of Nebraska College of Medicine
Nevada
   University of Nevada School of Medicine
New Hampshire
   Dartmouth Medical School
New Jersey
   New Jersey College of Medicine and Dentistry
   Rutgers—The State University—Rutgers Medical School
New Mexico
   University of New Mexico School of Medicine
New York
   Albany Medical College of Union University
   College of Physicians and Surgeons, Columbia University
   Cornell University Medical College
   Albert Einstein College of Medicine, Yeshiva University
   Mount Sinai School of Medicine

New York Medical College
New York University School of Medicine
University of Rochester School of Medicine and Dentistry
State University of New York at Buffalo School of Medicine
State University of New York Downstate Medical Center College of Medicine
State University of New York (Stony Brook) College of Medicine
State University of New York Upstate Medical Center College of Medicine
North Carolina
Bowman Gray School of Medicine of Wake Forest College
Duke University School of Medicine
University of North Carolina School of Medicine
North Dakota
University of North Dakota School of Medicine
Ohio
Case-Western Reserve University School of Medicine
University of Cincinnati College of Medicine
Medical College of Ohio at Toledo
Ohio State University College of Medicine
Oklahoma
University of Oklahoma School of Medicine
Oregon
University of Oregon Medical School
Pennsylvania
Hahnemann Medical College of Philadelphia
Jefferson Medical College of Philadelphia
University of Pennsylvania School of Medicine
Pennsylvania State University College of Medicine, Milton S. Hershey Medical Center
University of Pittsburgh School of Medicine
Temple University School of Medicine
Woman's Medical College of Pennsylvania
Rhode Island
Brown University Program in Medical Science
South Carolina
Medical College of South Carolina
South Dakota
University of South Dakota School of Medicine

Tennessee
Meharry Medical College School of Medicine
University of Tennessee College of Medicine
Vanderbilt University School of Medicine
Texas
Baylor University College of Medicine
University of Texas Medical Branch
University of Texas Medical School at San Antonio
University of Texas Southwestern Medical School
Utah
University of Utah College of Medicine
Vermont
University of Vermont College of Medicine
Virginia
Medical College of Virginia School of Medicine
University of Virginia School of Medicine
Washington
University of Washington School of Medicine
West Virginia
West Virginia University School of Medicine
Wisconsin
Marquette School of Medicine
University of Wisconsin Medical School

Affiliated Schools
Puerto Rico
University of Puerto Rico School of Medicine
Republic of the Philippines
University of the Philippines College of Medicine
Beirut, Lebanon
The American University of Beirut School of Medicine
Canada
University of Alberta Faculty of Medicine
University of Calgary Faculty of Medicine
University of British Columbia Faculty of Medicine
University of Manitoba Faculty of Medicine
Memorial University of Newfoundland
Dalhousie University Faculty of Medicine
McMaster University Faculty of Medicine
University of Ottawa Faculty of Medicine

Queen's University Faculty of Medicine
University of Toronto Faculty of Medicine
University of Western Ontario Faculty of Medicine
Universite Laval Faculte de Medecine
McGill University Faculty of Medicine
University de Montreal Faculte de Medecine
Universite de Sherbrooke Faculte de Medecine
University of Saskatchewan College of Medicine

Notes to Chapter Eight

1. *Medical School Admission Requirements,* 1968–1969, Association of American Medical Colleges. P. 252. Reprinted by permission.

Chapter Nine

FINANCIAL AID

Financial planning for the long-range goal of a medical education should begin in high school. With sufficient time to meet each obligation as it arises, the student with limited financial resources can plan to conserve and augment the amount of money he has available.

At the undergraduate level, part-time employment is possible. The student should not take on such a heavy work load, however, that he jeopardizes his academic performance, as admissions committees rely heavily on premedical grades as an indicator of probable success in medical school. Summer jobs and a controllable amount of work during the school year can contribute to premedical college expenses and to the building up of a reserve fund toward the medical education.

If possible, have sufficient funds on hand to cover your first year in college. College financial officers are much more willing to assist a student who is already enrolled and has begun to prove his academic ability than one who is unknown to them. This is often the case in medical school as well. Once enrolled, a student with a financial emergency will find that, the more credits he has completed, the greater access he has to private funds and scholarships.

Undergraduate Scholarships and Loans

From your junior year in high school, begin to work with your high school adviser and science teachers in planning to enter competitions and take scholarship examinations at the proper time, and to seek out sources of premedical financial aid. Even before the final decision regarding your college choice is made, you may be eligible for one of the national programs that offer scholarships to talented high school graduates by virtue of their academic records and participation in various competitions.

Details of some of the well-known programs can be obtained by writing to:

> Science Talent Search
> 1719 N Street, N.W.
> Washington, D. C. 20006
>
> National Honor Society
> National Association of Secondary School Principals
> 1201 Sixteenth St., N.W.
> Washington, D. C. 20006
>
> National Merit Scholarship Corporation
> 1580 Sherman Avenue
> Evanston, Illinois 60201

The Merit Program. The National Merit Scholarship Corporation's program is detailed here to illustrate how this type of honors program operates. The goals of the program include the identification of the talented student at an early level; Merit Scholars are those at the very top of the ability scale. A unique aspect of the program is the protection of the student's freedom of choice in selecting a college. The student is permitted to choose the college best suited to his academic and professional goals, no matter how expensive, and aid is awarded to implement this choice.

The merit program selects students according to their "developed ability and promise for future accomplishment, paying no attention to financial need." [1] Once they are selected, the amount of financial assistance given the winners is in direct relation to their actual needs in attending the colleges of their choice.

The spread of representative winners is across economic boundaries, although all must be high achievers. Any student aspiring to such an award should keep it in mind from the day he enters high school. Winners from families with incomes well above the national average receive a token $100 per year, plus the honor of being a Merit Scholar. Those from middle-income families receive annual amounts ranging from $400 to $950, depending on their individual requirements. Those from lower-income families receive the maximum stipend of $1,500 per year (or more in a few sponsored programs). Awards are four-year stipends to be used at the college of the recipient's choice.

A high school student enters the competition in the second semester of his junior year by taking the National Merit Scholarship Qualifying Test. On the basis of performance on this test, the highest scoring students in each state are named semifinalists. A semifinalist becomes eligible for a merit scholarship by attaining finalist status. To become a finalist, you must be endorsed by your high school, give an equivalent performance on a second test, supply grade records and information on academic and other honors, and provide family financial data to be used for computing the stipend if you are selected as a Merit Scholar. About 97 percent of the semifinalists become finalists. The Merit Scholars are selected from this group.

Achievement Program for Outstanding Negro Students. In 1964, a Ford Foundation grant of seven million dollars established a program independent of the merit program to identify, honor, and encourage superior academic attainment among Negro students. The grant underwrites two hundred scholarships a year over a five-year period; additional scholarships are underwritten by sponsors.

This achievement program consciously strives to encourage students at all levels of education to aim for higher goals of intellectual attainment. For younger students, it provides a goal toward which to work. Motivation of students has been one important result of the program. One high school counselor reported that many seniors who were not nominated expressed regret that they had not worked harder. In some areas, students have arranged speaking programs at junior high schools to tell the younger students that education does pay off and that they should make an early start on trying to get good grades.

Instead of the merit program's qualifying examination, finalists are selected from students nominated by school officials on the basis of grades, rank in class, honors, activities, and aspects of the student's character and personality that point to success in college and later in life. This method takes into consideration the talent loss that can occur from underdevelopment of intellectual abilities before the college years, particularly in the student from lower socioeconomic circumstances, who is less likely to enlarge his native gifts during his primary and secondary school years. For this reason, many talented Negroes were not reaching the talent pool of semifinalists in the regular merit program testing method of selection. The achievement program offsets this disadvantage.

The College Financial Aid Office. Once you have selected and applied to the college of your choice for your premedical studies, its office of financial aid is your best source of information on scholarships and loans. Most colleges have small grants or private funds available for students who qualify in one or more ways according to the stipulations of the donor. There are also emergency book funds, small emergency loan funds, and scholarships set up by local organizations and individuals, to assist students in a particular field or the children of members of the sponsoring organization. The individual colleges administer most government scholarship and loan programs for their students.

When you have been accepted by your college, inform the financial aid officer of your need for additional funds. You will usually be asked to complete an application for assistance, including a personal and family financial summary, for the use of the college in evaluating your needs and awarding the funds at its disposal.

A good student whose family's income is below ten thousand dollars annually can be eligible for a premedical scholarship ranging from two hundred dollars to two thousand dollars a year. Some of the sponsors of such scholarships are federal and state governments, local chapters of national fraternal organizations, drug companies, labor groups, fraternities and sororities, civic and service organizations, and individuals. Your local medical association is another source of information on scholarship and loan programs that may be available in your particular locality.

Work-Study Programs. Each college has a placement office that will assist students desirous of obtaining part-time, temporary, or summer employment. Many colleges also participate in the federally established College Work-Study Program. Most colleges, and often individual departments, have assistantships for students, who may work either in campus offices or in other campus jobs and facilities. Once you have selected your major subject and are in residence on campus, consult the chairman of that department about possible opportunities within the department. Department chairmen often know of funds established by private local sources for assisting needy students in a particular field or subject.

One note of caution in selecting on-campus employment: many of these jobs may not be the most practical means of earning extra money for a student who has a well-developed skill, who is a competent typist or laboratory technician, for instance. Estimate the hours required each week for a campus job or assistantship; and then compute an approximate hourly rate of pay. Often such work brings an average of seventy-five cents an hour. The student who can find off-campus employment at a higher rate would be well-advised to accept it, provided it fits into his class timetable and he has the necessary transportation.

Undergraduate Loan Programs. Colleges usually administer such loan programs as the National Defense Student Loan Program, under which needy college students with superior academic backgrounds receive special consideration. A premedical student can borrow up to one thousand dollars per year under this program.

Write for the current bulletin, *Federal Aids for College Students,* from the Office of Education, United States Department of Health, Education, and Welfare, Washington, D.C. 20202. This publication lists information on the College Student Guaranteed Loan Program. This program is administered differently in individual states—in some through an established state guarantee agency, in others through United Student Aid Funds, Inc., 845 Third Avenue, New York, New York 10022. Students may borrow up to one thousand dollars (fifteen hundred dollars in some states) toward undergraduate college expenses.

The Office of Education also publishes a pamphlet entitled *Get Ready for College and Go.* This is a guide to four programs of federal assistance in financing a college education: the College Work-Study Program; National Defense Student Loans; Educational Opportunity Grants (a program of direct awards of from two hundred dollars to eight hundred dollars per year to academically qualified students with exceptional financial need); and Guaranteed Loans (a program of borrowing for middle- and upper-income families who find a college education for their children a financial burden). This publication also contains a bibliography. In addition, the Office of Education recommends the American Legion's inexpensive publication, *Need A Lift?,* available at twenty-five cents per copy from Box 1055, Indianapolis, Indiana 46206.

The National Scholarship Service and Fund for Negro Students, 6 East 82nd Street, New York, New York 10028, maintains a counseling and referral college advisory service for high school students. Further information may be obtained from the organization.

The military services offer scholarships, loans, and grants to dependents of personnel on active duty, retired, or deceased. Specific information may be obtained from the various services. The offices and their addresses are listed in a newsletter, *Notes of Financial Aid for Students,* also published by the Office of Education.

For both scholarships and loans, consult some of the many reference books now available on the subject in the offices of guidance counselors and in school and public libraries, or order copies for your personal use from the publishers. The College Entrance Examination Board recommends *Scholarships, Fellowships and Loans,* by S. Norman Feingold, Bellman Publishers, Cambridge, Massachusetts.[2] An excellent bibliography of financial aid publications is contained in the reprint, *Career Information for High School Students,* which can be obtained from the Association of American Medical Colleges, 2530 Ridge Avenue, Evanston, Illinois 60201.

Horizons Unlimited also contains a reading list with a section on publications pertaining to the financing of a college or medical education. This book is available in the offices of guidance counselors or from the American Medical Association, 535 North Dearborn Street, Chicago, Illinois 60610.

Financing Medical School Education

Students should not rely on part-time work during medical school, particularly in the preclinical years. Many physicians point out that, by not working during medical school, they were able to earn top grades and qualify more readily for scholarships.

Dr. James Bartlett, of the University of Rochester, agrees with this theory, and goes even further. "We advise our medical students not to work during the semester. I like to see them take a few hundred more in a loan. We do not want them to invest their extra time in work. Recreation and relaxation are more important during this time."

Again, if a student can amass sufficient reserves to carry him through the first year of medical school, he will discover more and more sources of financial aid available to him as he progresses through school. Families who understand this situation should be encouraged to avail themselves of the many loan programs now open to help finance medical school tuition. In many instances, families who are willing, and even eager, to assume debts to finance a son in medical school are reluctant to do so for a daughter. Instead, they try to talk their girls out of such ambitions. It is up to the young woman to convince her family of the sincerity of her motivation and to enlist their support, particularly for the early stages of her medical education.

Medical School Costs. Medical school tuition and costs are high, but the cost range is wide. The lowest estimates of minimum annual expenses are given by tax-supported schools for their first-year resident students (all figures given are median): tuition, $618; room and board, $1,000; books and supplies, $212. The comparable nonresident public school tuition fee is $1,220; room, board, and other expenses are the same.

Private schools are more costly, and the range is even wider. Tuition and fees begin at a minimum of $1,068 and go to a maximum of $2,595, with a median figure of $1,930 per year. Median estimates at a private institution for room and board are $1,200, and for books and supplies $200.[3]

In addition to the above expenses, the student should be prepared to furnish himself with a microscope. Before purchasing one, consult the school you will be attending for detailed information on the type of instrument required. Most schools now require as minimum equipment a monocular microscope with four objectives. A binocular instrument is better if you can afford the higher price; it also reduces fatigue and eyestrain.

Monocular microscopes manufactured in the United States range from about $400 to $750; binocular start at about $700 and go as high as $1,100. Less expensive microscopes, including many reputable foreign makes, are acceptable at some schools. Used microscopes are often available through medical schools at greatly reduced prices. You should know that many schools require official approval of used microscopes (and often of new ones). This is especially important in the case of used instruments, which may have mechanical or optical faults or features of obsolescence easily overlooked by anyone unfamiliar with them.

Scholarships Awarded by Medical Schools. Each medical school has its own funds for scholarships and grants. The financial aid office of the medical school at which you have been accepted is the place to begin seeking sources of assistance. Both public and private schools award scholarships on the basis of scholastic performance and financial need, the size of the award being determined by the latter.

The Health Professions Scholarship Program. The Health Professions Scholarship Program, authorized by the government in 1965, is designed to enable talented students who do not have the necessary funds to enter the health professions. "These scholarships are available only to students who, without the amount of the scholarship award, could not pursue the required studies at such schools during the year for which the award is made." [4] In order to qualify for this assistance, a student must be from a low-income family.

The scholarships are administered by the medical schools themselves, which select all the recipients. The maximum amount you may receive under this program each year is $2,500. In determining the amount of the scholarship, the school will consider the total expenses of attending school for a year and the financial resources available to you for meeting those expenses. No student need ever say again that he could not attend medical school *only* because he was the victim of limited financial resources. The Public Health Service (Washington, D. C. 20201) has a folder available describing the program, but application forms must be obtained from the scholarship office of the school in which you expect to enroll.

State Scholarships. Many states offer scholarship grants to their residents to pursue a medical education. Contact your state's board of education to see if such a program exists and what the requirements for eligibility are. An example of such a program is the New York State Regents Scholarship for Medicine and Dentistry, which is awarded on a competitive basis to college students who reside in the state. Residents may also apply for the New York State Scholar Incentive Program, which offers individual awards of one hundred dollars to four hundred dollars per semester. Awards are based on the taxable income of the parents and on tuition costs.

Many states have programs of financial aid that "forgive" part or all of the money awarded if the student practices medicine in that state after completing his training. If the student decides to practice elsewhere, repayment is required. An example of this type of program is the one administered by the Medical Education Board of Georgia to aid resident students and to provide medical services to rural areas. Awards are made of up to $1,250 per year; for each year of service in rural Georgia, $1,000 of the award is forgiven.

State and county medical associations are also sources of scholarship aid. These scholarships average about one thousand dollars per year and are available to local students going to medical school. Some carry the stipulation that the student practice in a particular area of need upon graduation, or repay part or all of the funds granted. Others simply carry a moral obligation to repay the source area in service. Such is the program established by the Committee on Rural Health of the Ohio State Medical Association, which awards scholarships only to men and women from small Ohio communities. It is hoped that these students, familiar with the problems of rural areas, will later practice in such areas.

Many private foundations, religious organizations, business firms, and pharmaceutical houses provide scholarship aid to eligible students. Some restrict their aid to members of the organization and/or their families. Others sponsor worthy students who are residents of the area in which the sponsoring organization is located. The publication *Medical School Admission Requirements* lists representative sources of such aid and includes a bibliography on further sources of financial aid.

Aid to Minority Groups. The National Medical Fellowships organization was established to provide assistance to Negroes for education and training in medicine. Scholarships and grants-in-aid for undergraduate medical study are awarded to talented Negro men and women who are United States citizens and have been admitted to medical school. Grants are offered for a period of one academic year and are renewable. They are awarded on the basis of academic performance and financial need.

In addition to the annual awards, in 1968 ten outstanding Negro college students were awarded four-year medical scholarships, averaging eight thousand dollars each, under the National Medical-Sloan Foundation scholarship program. Of the 544 Negroes who have received financial support from National Medical Fellowships since its inception in 1946, about 10 percent have been women. Further details and application blanks may be obtained from: Executive Secretary, National Medical Fellowships, Inc., 3935 Elm Street, Downers Grove, Illinois 60515. The deadline for the receipt of completed applications each year is March 1.

Another organization dedicated to the assistance of students from minority groups is the John Hay Whitney Foundation, 111 West 50th Street, New York, New York 10020. Each year, this foundation makes two to four awards in the field of medicine, up to a maximum grant of three thousand dollars for the full academic year. Competition is open to American citizens of Negro, Spanish-American, and American Indian backgrounds and to citizens who are residents of the southern Appalachian and Ozark mountain areas, Guam, Puerto Rico, Samoa, Pacific Trust Territory, and the Virgin Islands.

Local Scholarship Funds. Individual medical schools usually have scholarship funds established by many and varied local sources, including individuals, memorial funds, clubs and organizations, businesses, and foundations. These funds may be endowments provided for deserving students in need of financial help, to be awarded at the discretion of the college administration, or special sums to be awarded to students with specific eligibility requirements. Many doctors and organizations establish prizes for achievement in certain fields of study. The student will find that many of these sources become available to him once he is enrolled and attending medical school. Often, the aid is reserved for second-year or clinical students who have proven their ability in their medical studies. The individual medical schools can provide detailed information on the scholarship funds at their disposal.

Loan Programs. The Federal Health Professions Student Loan Program provides financial assistance to medical students in the form of long-term loans. Administration of the loan funds is the responsibility of the medical schools. No loans are made directly to students by the federal government. Students must be able to demonstrate that they need the loan in order to pursue their courses of study.

The maximum amount a student may borrow for an academic year is $2,500. A loan *may* be made at any time during the year if the student can demonstrate that he needs it to complete the school year. The medical school will consider the total expenses of school attendance during the year and the other financial resources available to the student when determining the amount of the loan.[5]

The loans are repayable to the school over a ten-year period, beginning three years after completion or cessation of the prescribed full-time course of study. Interest charges begin at the time the loan becomes repayable. Loan deferments can be arranged up to a maximum of three years for active duty in the armed services or in the Peace Corps.

Loan applications should be obtained from the participating medical school; they are *not* available from the Public Health Service. Students participating in this program are ineligible for the National Defense Student Loan Fund.

A portion of a Federal Health Professions Student Loan can be repaid in service after the student has completed his training. The Health Professions Educational Assistance Act authorizes forgiveness of up to 50 percent (10 percent annually) of the amount of a loan, plus accrued interest, for the student who subsequently practices in an area certified as having a shortage of health personnel under regulations drawn up by the Department of Health, Education, and Welfare.

Up to 100 percent of the amount of the loan (plus interest) that is unpaid as of the first day of the borrower's medical practice may be canceled, at the rate of 15 percent for each complete year of practice, if he works in a rural shortage area characterized by low family incomes.

By writing to the Office of Education, U.S. Department of Health, Education, and Welfare, Washington, D. C. 20202, in care of the Division of Student Financial Aid, you can obtain a booklet, *Aids to Students,* which describes all the Health Professions scholarship and loan programs and provides valuable career information.

Another major program of financial assistance is the American Medical Association's Medical Education Loan Guarantee Program. Through this program, banks are enabled to provide loans for medical students, interns, and residents in good standing who are enrolled in full-time training at an American medical school or hospital approved by the Council on Medical Education of the AMA. To qualify, students must have completed their first semester or quarter of medical school and must be citizens of the United States.

A substantial portion of the cost of a medical education can be financed through this program. The funds to back up the bank loans are contributed by organizations, corporations, and individuals. As much as fifteen hundred dollars may be borrowed annually, and a maximum total of ten thousand dollars may be borrowed over a period of seven years. The student's total educational loans from *all* sources may not exceed fifteen thousand dollars.

A medical student may submit no more than one loan application each academic quarter or semester. Interns and residents may not submit more than one application every six months. The minimum amount of a loan is four hundred dollars, and loans must be in even multiples of one hundred dollars. Medical students who desire information about these loans should contact the dean's office of their school.

The interest rates on the AMA-Education and Research Foundation-sponsored loans are higher than on government loans but lower than on personal bank loans. The current (1968) agreement with the banks provides for a maximum ten-year repayment period, with simple interest of 7 percent. The rate in effect at the time a given note is signed will remain unchanged during the entire life of that loan. If a student borrows several times during his training period, some of the notes may carry different interest rates than others, due to fluctuations in the prime rate. An interim note is executed for each individual loan.

To apply for a loan, obtain application forms from your medical school dean's office and complete two copies of the application (AMA-ERF 102). Next, secure and complete a copy of the interim note (AMA-ERF 103). Obtain certification of the application from the dean (or from the program director or chief of service, as applicable). Finally, mail all the completed materials to the participating bank of your choice.[6]

The American Medical Women's Association has a loan program for women medical students who are United States citizens and are enrolled in accredited United States medical schools. The maximum amount that may be borrowed is one thousand dollars per year; interest of 4 percent per annum begins six months after graduation. Application should be made to the association at 1740 Broadway, New York, New York 10019. A personal interview is required; the AMWA will designate a physician who resides in the applicant's area.

Private corporations, unions, and fraternal and service organizations are also sources of loan assistance. Some restrict participation to employees and their children. For example, the General Electric Company has educational loans available for children of GE employees. Parents must apply for the loans through the company. Maximum loans of one thousand dollars per year are available.

United Student Aid Funds, Inc., 845 Third Avenue, New York, New York 10022, is a national nonprofit loan program established to endorse low-cost commercial loans for full-time graduate students. The maximum that may be borrowed is $1,500 per year. The student must apply through his medical school, since the participating school recommends the loan. The student's local bank handles the loan on the student's own signature. Repayment begins nine months after graduation from medical or graduate school.

State and local medical societies, state governments, and public and private foundations have loan programs, and the student should follow basically the same procedure in seeking information about these as he would with scholarship assistance. The individual medical schools have loan funds, some for long-term financing and smaller emergency funds for short-term borrowing. Again, the medical school is your source for details concerning what is available.

State, local, and regional aid is often directed to those students who plan to practice in the area providing the funds. Residents who qualify can receive aid, and often the greater portion of the loan is forgiven if the student signs a contract to practice for a certain length of time in a stipulated area. Residents of states that have loan programs for medical students can secure details of such programs from the state board of education.

Postgraduate Financial Assistance

Internship, residency, and postgraduate research can also be financed through grants and loans if necessary. Although interns and residents can usually meet most of their expenses from their salaries, supplemental funds may occasionally be needed.

Many of the specialty boards provide funds to residents training in that particular specialty. Some of the opportunities available have been mentioned in the preceding chapters pertaining to internship and residency. The Association of American Medical Colleges publishes a book titled *Financial Assistance Available for Graduate Study in Medicine,* which can be obtained from the association at Evanston, Illinois 60201. The association's *Medical School Admission Requirements,* mentioned previously, also contains listings of representative postgraduate aid.

Students who intend to pursue research careers in the medical or physical sciences will find a wealth of research fellowships, funds, and prizes to support their investigations. The National Science Foundation has fellowship programs, and a substantial number of awards (about one-fourth) have thus far been made to women. Women in the life sciences—that is, biochemistry, general biology, and microbiology—have received considerable support in their graduate work. Women have also won about one-fifth of the fellowships granted each year by the National Institutes of Health.[7]

The guaranteed, long-term bank loan program of the American Medical Association's Education and Research Foundation also applies to postgraduate training. Interns and residents who are United States citizens in full-time training and good standing may borrow up to $750 per year for their living and training expenses. Application should be made through your hospital administrator's office or chief of service. (*See* previous section on loan programs for medical school for application procedures.)

National Medical Fellowships, Inc., continues its support of promising Negro physicians into their postgraduate training. While its scholarships go only to undergraduate medical students, Negro physicians may obtain loans of up to $1,500 per year, with repayment beginning no later than three years after completion of training.

The Radcliffe Institute, 78 Mount Auburn Street, Cambridge, Massachusetts 02138, has fellowships funded by the Josiah Macy, Jr., Foundation for woman medical students and postgraduate scholars. The funds may be applied to either part-time or full-time study or training, and the money can be used for any and all expenses, including child care and household help. A detailed description of this excellent program, which takes into consideration the special needs of a woman in the medical profession, is to be found in Part III of this book.

The National Association of Interns and Residents, Inc., 41 East 42nd Street, New York, New York 10017, has an emergency loan fund for its members. An intern or resident can borrow up to two hundred dollars at no interest. The association also provides four annual grants of five hundred dollars each for special postgraduate study projects.

Notes to Chapter Nine

1. *The Merit Program: The First Decade,* National Merit Scholarship Corporation, Evanston, Ill., 1966.
2. Personal communication from William D. Van Dusen, Assistant Director, College Scholarship Service, College Entrance Examination Board, New York, N.Y., November 30, 1966.
3. *Medical School Admission Requirements,* 1968–69, American Association of Medical Colleges. Ch. 4, table 4.2, pp. 29, 30. Reprinted by permission.
4. *The Health Professions Scholarship Program,* Public Health Service, U.S. Department of Health, Education, and Welfare, 1968.

5. *The Health Professions Student Loan Program*, Public Health Service, U.S. Department of Health, Education, and Welfare, 1968.
6. *Medical Education Loan Guarantee Program*, American Medical Association, 1968.
7. *Women in Scientific Careers*, National Science Foundation, 1961.

Chapter Ten

MEDICAL SCHOOL

What is medical school really like? How do the students manage? What do the courses cover? Could *I* complete medical school successfully? Every girl considering a medical career asks herself these and similar questions, but very few have the opportunity to find out the answers by seeing the inside of a medical school during the important high school years when career preparation should begin.

"It's worse than I thought it would be!" one girl admitted candidly, after finishing her sophomore year in medical school. "This is the first time in my life I ever had to buckle down and cram to make a 'C.' "

And yet, despite the rugged schedule, the enormous texts that must be read and digested, the constant preparation for quizzes and exams, and the lack of sleep, the girls interviewed felt equal to the task. They rarely complained of the actual curriculum, seemed absorbed in what they were studying, and described with enthusiasm their medical school experience to any interested listener. The frequency of tests seemed to be the biggest gripe.

"I wish they would do away with grading and the 'curve' system," said one. "Competition is cutthroat all around; girls are not exempt."

The first- and second-year programs consist of classes, labs, seminars, and conferences from 9 A.M. to 5 P.M., five days a week. There are few or no electives at this level, and there is very little free time. The first two years are the worst, most medical students agree; once you've cleared this hurdle, you're on your way.

Following is a summary of the typical curriculum offered in most medical schools, with a general description of the course material. It is in no way intended to be a complete schedule or a description of the only type of curriculum available, but is a sample drawn from the announcement bulletins of medical schools in different parts of the country.

The Preclinical Years

During the first two years of medical school, the course of instruction is concentrated lecture and laboratory work, plus research in the medical library. Students learn the normal, and then the abnormal, structure and functions of the human body and personality. Studies in the preclinical years center on the basic medical sciences, summarized below.

Anatomy. The anatomy of the human body is studied on both the gross (visible to the naked eye) and microscopic levels, with emphasis on correlation of structure and function. Gross anatomy consists of laboratory dissection of a human cadaver, supported by lectures and conferences. Cell biology includes the study of the correlation of cellular structure and function, with laboratory observation of slides under the light microscope. The following subjects are studied both in the laboratory and in lectures: Histology deals with the light and electron microscopy of systems and organs. Neuroanatomy deals with the development and organization of the central nervous system. Genetics is the study of heredity—the genetic control of, and the fundamental processes in, development.

Biochemistry. Courses include the study of the structure and chemical properties of cellular and tissue components; metabolism and biosynthesis of carbohydrates, lipids, proteins, steroids, porphyrins, and nucleic acids; and the role of enzymes and hormones in the regulation of metabolism. Systemic biochemistry deals with the functioning of the circulatory, respiratory, excretory, nervous, digestive, and endocrine systems. The course material is presented in lectures, conferences, and laboratory work.

Pathology. General pathology familiarizes the student with the structural and functional manifestations of disease and their relevance to diagnosis, pathogenesis, and therapy. Lectures stress basic mechanisms; laboratory instruction includes examination of microscopic slides and the study of gross organ pathology. Special pathology utilizes the concepts of general pathology in an intensive study of human disease by organ systems. By means of seminars, visual aids, and autopsy pathology, the pathological observations in a disease state are related to clinical problems.

Physiology. This science is the study of the functions of organs and parts of the body during life. The subjects covered include general biophysical principles as related to cellular physiology, especially those of nerve and muscle; the structural and functional relationships in the cardiovascular system; excretory functions; gastro-intestinal and endocrine systems; and digestion. The course material is presented in lectures, laboratory work, and conferences.

Microbiology. This science includes basic bacteriology, genetics of microorganisms, biochemistry and physiology of microorganisms, and their application to clinical medicine. Course work emphasizes the diagnosis and control of infectious diseases caused by bacteria, spirochetes, rickettsiae, viruses, and fungi.

Pharmacology. In pharmacology, the science of drugs, basic pharmacological principles and the special pharmacology of important organ systems are introduced. The study of toxicology, therapeutic drugs used in the treatment of infections, the concepts of allergy, the toxic action of important drugs and poisons, and prescription writing are also part of the course work.

Other subjects studied. In addition to the above basic medical sciences, courses in clinical pathology and laboratory analysis, physical diagnosis and history-taking, biostatistics, preventive medicine, psychiatry, and radiology are also taken in the first two years.

As soon as preliminary instruction permits, students begin the examination of healthy persons and of patients, under the close supervision of faculty members.

There are opportunities to pursue individual research projects in the various departments. Supervised research is often available to medical students during the summer term, or on a part-time basis during the regular academic year. Selected students may pursue additional studies in the subjects of their special interest in many of the research laboratories of the medical school.

Budgeting Your Time in the Preclinical Years. "The biggest problem for me is getting everything done that I have to do. Most of the girls in my class want to learn thoroughly . . . conscientiously, and we don't always have the time to do it. You really have to budget your time and stick to it. You *must* study."

A diminutive, brunette, second-year medical student at the University of Miami (Florida), Leslie Polland regrets her delayed start in medicine. She came to it via the route of laboratory technician, working and studying part-time for several years before deciding to enter medical school. While working in the lab, she attended college in the evening, but found the progress so slow that she decided to finish her college work on a full-time basis. She quit her job, completed the ninety-credit premed minimum, and entered medical school the following year.

"I assumed you had to be a genius to become a doctor. My concept of a physician was of complete dedication; [I believed] it was necessary to devote one's whole life to medicine. Most women don't know there are plenty of jobs in the profession where you can work from nine to five. Had I known this, I would have gone into medicine directly from high school."

The old refrain . . . "if only I had known, I would have decided earlier." The most consistent encouragement women in medicine can offer to those thinking about becoming doctors is, "Don't put off your decision—you *can* do it."

This ambitious student is self-supporting, without a scholarship or much family assistance. Leslie works one night a week at a nearby hospital; her earnings there completely pay for her room and board. She earns the bulk of her tuition money in the laboratory of another local hospital, working two or three shifts per week, depending upon the study load. "On holidays, I work the whole day to pick up spending money. My parents also send me about two hundred dollars a year."

She admits such a schedule can wreak havoc with a girl's social calendar, but has found an agreeable compromise.

"I date like crazy in the summer and then cut down on dates during the school term. I must study six hours a night every weeknight, and this keeps me so busy that I don't miss outside activities. Weekend nights are strictly for parties, fun, and ice-skating at a nearby indoor rink with a group of the medical students. If you don't go out and have fun each week, you become bitter and . . . study inefficiently. On Sunday, I just relax in the sun—don't open a book. I need the safety valve of a day completely without study."

The American Medical Association stresses a well-rounded personality as one of the elements for success in medicine. Leslie not only concurs but has a high regard for her fellow classmates:

"I was amazed at how many of the girls sew—I mean design their own patterns and everything. A reason for this could be the high level of creativity of medical students. People who go into medicine have so many talents that they could go into many other fields successfully. They paint, sculpt . . . and most of the men play musical instruments."

Don't budget your time so rigidly that you eliminate your favorite leisure pursuits. Creative activities and simple relaxation are as important to your equanimity as an effective study regime.

The Clinical Years

Junior and senior medical students concentrate less on theory and more on the actual practice of medicine. The doctor-patient relationship becomes increasingly important during the clinical years. Most of the student's time is spent in the hospital wards, working under the guidance of faculty members who supervise the taking of patient histories, physical examinations, case studies, diagnosis, and follow-ups.

The clinical experience is augmented by lectures, laboratory work, record keeping, and seminars.

Students rotate through the services described below to complete their *core clerkships.* They participate in ward and clinic work, conferences, and case presentations. The upperclassmen make ward rounds for observation, make tentative diagnoses under the supervision of hospital staff and faculty members, and in seminars present and defend their diagnoses and prescribed therapy. Each student becomes familiar with all the patients on the service, but works closely with only a certain number that are assigned to him.

"The underlying aim of clinical training is to present the principles and practices of medical care so that the student acquires a basic understanding of his patients as total human beings." [1]

Medicine. Students develop their skills in physical diagnosis and history-taking. They are responsible for complete histories, initiate diagnostic investigations, and discuss cases with a faculty tutor who is responsible for the work of only two to four students.

In the fourth year, the student is assigned patients who are admitted to the hospital affiliated with the medical school, and he follows their progress throughout their hospitalization. He now participates fully in planning the diagnostic investigation and treatment of his patients. He attends conferences and seminars held by the various subspecialty sections of the department of medicine.

The student also receives instruction in the medical specialty fields, such as dermatology, neurology, ophthalmology, otolaryngology, and urology.

Obstetrics and Gynecology. The clinical course in obstetrics and gynecology consists of lectures, seminars, demonstrations, and care of outpatient cases. The course material covers pathology, complications of pregnancy, labor, and other important gynecological topics. Instruction in these subjects is given to small groups of students.

Fourth-year students are assigned to the hospital for supervised clinical experience, including assistance in the delivery room; in some cases, a student may officiate at a normal delivery.

Pediatrics. Third-year students are introduced to the main concerns of pediatrics, growth and development, the processes that enable the child to achieve his full potential physically, mentally, emotionally, and socially. The students are then assigned to sick children in the wards and in the outpatient clinic. Under close supervision, they study each patient's history and take part in his physical examination, diagnosis, treatment, and prognosis.

Surgery. Lectures and demonstrations in the basic principles of surgery are presented during the sophomore year. More advanced study of general surgery is pursued in the third year, with participation in group conferences and seminars. The students then are assigned to the department of surgery at the affiliated hospital for supervised clinical experience designed to integrate general surgery with the medical specialties, psychiatry, and radiology.

Fourth-year students, working under constant supervision, are responsible for assigned patients from admission to discharge. The students record complete histories of their patients, perform physical examinations, order indicated laboratory and X-ray studies, request consultations, and present the problems to their consultants. The students also attend regular departmental conferences and student surgical conferences for evaluation and discussion of selected cases. They scrub up and serve on the team of assistants in the operating room.

Psychiatry. Under faculty supervision, third-year students interview patients and study the basic concepts of psychiatric history-taking and the determination of mental status. The lectures in psychiatry deal with the management of neuroses, psychoses, and psychiatric emergencies. The students also participate in clinic work, ward rounds, and medical panels.

Fourth-year students are assigned to psychiatric clinical duties at the affiliated hospital, under close faculty and staff supervision. They follow their patients' progress through hospital admission, treatment, and discharge. The major psychosomatic and psychiatric disorders are observed in the course of ward rounds, demonstrations, and case presentations. Students also gain experience in child psychiatry and often participate in group psychotherapy sessions.

Clinical Training Methods. The only preparation for clinical medicine that most third-year students have had is an introductory course in physical diagnosis. At the beginning of the third year, they are assigned to ward teams of the various clinical services, comprising the resident staff, an intern, two students (usually a junior and a senior), and the attending physician. The latter is the faculty member responsible for everything that happens on the ward in his service. During the junior year, the students complete the core clerkships described above. Usually, they also complete shorter services in neurology and anesthesiology.

Rounds are one of the primary teaching methods for training physicians. The ward team goes from bed to bed, discussing the patients' progress, an activity that takes most of the morning every day. Students make presentations and recommendations, but they do not prescribe until they have their M.D.'s. Once a week, each department has "grand rounds" of case presentations and discussion.

The bedside approach to teaching involves much participation in small group conferences. The students meet with a faculty member for three or four seminars a week. Interesting cases are discussed in detail, and pathological problems are studied. The conferences are under the direction of clinical faculty members and attending physicians from the voluntary faculty. In some services, a small group of students (from three to six) are assigned to a physician for instruction in his particular specialty.

A gradual, step-by-step increase in responsibility occurs from the third year in medical school through internship. Senior students carry more responsibility on the ward team; they function much like interns. It is the incremental assumption of responsibility, rather than any change of duties, that characterizes seniority. "Everybody teaches," one dean stated. "It is remarkable what you can learn from a student!"

The student works closely with patients from the beginning of his third year. In surgery, the student is probably closer to the patient than anyone else on the ward team. One attending physician remembers the afternoon he stopped by to tell a patient that his surgery had been scheduled for the following morning. The patient answered hesitantly, "Well, all right, but first I'd like to talk it over with my doctor." The "doctor" he was referring to was the student who had been assigned to his case—his surgeon was standing right in front of him.

Students in the clinical years are examined in their clinical abilities several times. One school's department of medicine, for example, gives four examinations on the wards during the student's tour of the service. For each test, a different examiner goes with the student to a patient's bedside while the student takes the history and arrives at a diagnosis. The doctor observes the student's skill, organization, and ability to discuss symptoms, and evaluates his diagnosis of the case and suggestions for therapy. Such examinations test the student's ability as a physician, rather than his facility at remembering facts in a book.

Within the last two years, almost every medical school in the United States has gone through the upheaval of a curriculum revision. The trend is toward more flexibility in selection of clerkships in the senior year and more free electives at the lower levels of instruction. Several medical schools now have a fourth year completely composed of electives, enabling students to explore the services and subspecialties that interest them in more depth. A person interested in a specialty can concentrate on that, taking only one or two services and their phases, or he can sample a wider range of specialties, such as cardiology, ear-nose-throat, radiology, and other selected services.

"This senior program of electives is the coming thing," one dean explained enthusiastically. "Until recently medicine had the most rigidly structured curriculum of any discipline. Now we are trying to introduce a wider range of flexibility to suit individual needs. The student now has the option to plan his own program to gain the experience suited to his particular interest."

Attitudes Toward Women in Medical School

Currently, only 9 percent of the students enrolled in medical schools in the United States are women. How, in the opinion of these young ladies, does their feminine identity hold up in an almost totally masculine environment? What are the attitudes of their male peers toward woman medical students?

Most of the women interviewed said they felt no discrimination at all toward them because of their sex. Although there is still some reluctance on the part of admissions committees to accept women because of the fear that they will not use their education as much as men will, this attitude affects neither the actual rate of acceptance nor the treatment of the female students once admitted. About half of the women who apply find seats in medical school; about half of the male applicants are also accepted.[2]

"I don't think there are enough bright girls in medical school. I see some girls who have been accepted only because, I think, they are girls. Most medical schools want to have a few girls in each class nowadays, and if women applied in greater numbers, they would be accepted. Intelligent girls do not apply in anywhere near the numbers that men do. Pretty girls get a lot of attractive offers . . . it is so easy to get detoured along the way." —Dr. Libby Connor, *Clinical Faculty, Jackson Memorial Hospital.*

The Macy Foundation, in evaluating its three-year-old program, Women for Medicine, has found that the medical school environment today is more receptive to women than in the past.

"The day of the hostile male student is passing. Seventy-five percent of our male medical students are married. They have domestic responsibilities, and they are more mature in their relationships with women. They understand what it is like to live with a woman; they see her as a wife and a mother. The 'domestication' of the male medical student in the United States has introduced a changing attitude in our male students toward women."[3]

Do male medical students make a practice of dating their female classmates? How do the girls feel they rate as women, apart from their desire to be accepted as competent professionals?

Dr. Helen Glaser, who conducted a questionnaire survey of female medical students, reported at the Macy Conference on Women for Medicine that many girls in her sample believed it was definitely an advantage to be a woman in medical school. They believed that, because of their sex, they enjoyed more pleasant treatment from both fellow students and faculty than was accorded the male students. Those who maintained a distinctly feminine role found that being a woman in a predominantly male community was a source of enjoyment.

The women in the Glaser sample who had complaints felt that they were singled out by their instructors, that their errors were more easily noticed and remembered, and that every failure on their part was ascribed to their sex.[4]

Carol Lopate found that the girls she interviewed tended to divide themselves into two groups: those who joined in a type of "buddy-buddy casual relationship with the opposite sex" and those who sat with other girls in classes, labs, and at meals, and generally were willing to identify with those of their own sex.[5]

The greatest concern of the woman students is to maintain their feminine identity in a predominantly male environment, while competing academically with their male colleagues. Some of the girls have moments (and for a few—months) of loneliness. Others find they have to develop considerable tact and make a conscious effort not to appear to show up the men in their classes. As one intern put it: "It isn't good for a woman to have her hand up first with the right answer. I am not sure that this is right. It may reflect social standards that are imposed on us and accepted while we are in medical school." [6]

None of the many students interviewed for this book admitted to feeling the pressure of competition between the sexes. The girls emphasized that "if you act like a lady, they treat you like a lady." While several belonged to the "buddy-buddy" group, they too were dating their classmates and every one of them felt accepted as a student, not condescendingly as "only a girl." Many said openly that they enjoyed the status quo and were satisfied socially. Several admitted that the competition for grades was "cutthroat" in the preclinical years, but they did not believe that being a woman made any difference in the way they were treated in class. Competition existed, but it was student versus student, not man versus woman.

"There have been some men who didn't like me," one dynamic blonde laughed. "I don't think it was because I was a girl in medicine. They wouldn't have liked me outside of medical school, either."

Some of the men's attitudes toward women in medical school are summarized below:

"How do our men feel about the girls in their classes? Ha—they marry them!" laughed one admissions officer.

"The field used to attract women who could not make it in the social world; that is now almost gone. Most women now are entering the field for sincere motives rather than because they do not see themselves as wives. In medical school, the male students treated us like royalty. I dated many of my fellow students, and so did the other four girls in my class. In fact, we girls dated them almost to the point of extinction from medical school."—*Graduate, Cornell University School of Medicine.*

Leslie Polland, of the University of Miami, finds that a girl's position in medical school is all too equal. She believes the attitudes of the men toward the woman students is neither antagonistic nor helpful: "You are treated completely as an equal. They do not open doors for you . . . you do not open doors for them. You are on your own completely."

Cathy Tullsen, of the University of Rochester, disagreed about this one point from her own experience. At Rochester, at least, men still open doors for women and recognize femininity. "I date the other students and am going out more than I did in college. And . . . the parties are the greatest!"

Dr. Lenor Zies, a recent graduate of the University of Miami School of Medicine (whose story is told in Chapter Twelve), summed up what turned out to be the consensus of female student opinion:

"How the men accept you depends on you. I always try to look and act like a girl, and they treat me like a girl. Even now that I am interning, I get up a half hour earlier than necessary to put makeup on and tease my hair. I did this in medical school, too, even if I had a test that day.

"I like to look my best all the time—it gives me a lift on a busy day when a patient asks how I can look so well at 5:00 A.M. I always keep my shoes clean, my person and makeup fresh; I don't use coarse language. It all takes some time and trouble, but I think it is worth the effort.

"Many girls are still playing the old part; some try to act more like men, ignoring makeup and feminine ways, and the men as a result don't treat them like ladies. I always dated the other students in medical school and married one of my classmates."

The other side of the story was presented by a dean of admissions at a school that is—despite his cautious attitude—quite liberal in its acceptance of woman students.

"A medical student has to work very hard. The curriculum of a medical school requires a person's complete time and attention. I am not for marriage being combined with medical school, from the experience I have observed here. We just recently accepted a young woman who was married last winter to a businessman. Is that businessman going to be willing to follow her here from a distant state while she attends our school?

"Another girl entered our school three years ago, married to a professional man—not a physician, however. During the evaluation and interview, I talked with her husband. At that time, he said there was nothing better he could think of for his wife than for her to pursue a career in medicine. The marriage has now ended in divorce, although she is a successful student and entering her last year. But I am not willing to break up a marriage just to get a medical student."

The almost unanimous conclusion of students, faculty, physicians, and admissions officers, based on their conglomerate experience, is that romance at the dating level and a happy, active social life are quite compatible with the study of medicine as long as a girl uses common sense and responsibility in planning her time and managing her studies.

Marriage is a different animal. The girl with the least chance of success, according to the women interviewed, is the one who, before entering medical school, has married someone outside the medical profession. The husband has to be willing to follow his wife to medical school. Doing so may affect his business or profession, and certainly will put strains on the marriage.

The longer a girl is in medical school, the better seem her chances for success with the career-marriage combination. When the difficult preclinical years are out of the way, she will have more time to devote to a husband and family. Also she will be more likely to choose a mate in the profession, one who understands the demands on her time and energies, one who may be going through the same problems himself and will be a sympathetic helpmate. Marriages between classmates or between woman medical students and young physicians seem to work out the best.

A man who marries a woman doctor must be much more secure in his career or profession and in his own intelligence than the average male. As Dr. Libby Connor sums it up:

"I always said before I married that I would not marry a doctor because you'd get so wrapped up in medicine that you'd think and talk nothing else. But you marry whom you meet, and of course all I met were doctors. So my husband is also a physician. I do think there are very few men who will marry a woman who makes them feel her career is more important than her man. A woman can make a go of both her marriage and medicine if she thinks of home as her primary responsibility and lets her man know it."

Notes to Chapter Ten

1. *Medical School Admission Requirements, 1968–69,* Association of American Medical Colleges, 1968. P. 39. Reprinted by permission.
2. *Journal of the American Medical Association,* Vol. 198, No. 8, November 21, 1966. Figures and comparisons also made from same study published in 1965: Davis G. Johnson, Ph.D., "The Study of Applicants, 1964–1965," *Journal of Medical Education,* Vol. 40, November, 1965.
3. *Report for the Year 1967,* Josiah Macy, Jr., Foundation. P. 53.
4. Carol Lopate, *Women in Medicine,* Johns Hopkins Press, 1968. Pp. 81–83.
5. *Ibid.*
6. *Ibid.*

Chapter Eleven

FOREIGN STUDY AND OPPORTUNITIES TO PRACTICE ABROAD

Whatever the motives for wanting to study medicine abroad, the student who plans to return to the United States to practice should be aware of the difficulties he will encounter upon his return. A student who seeks acceptance to a foreign medical school because of a low academic average in his undergraduate studies or a low MCAT score will find it difficult, and in many cases impossible, to pass the required tests and obtain licensing in this country, even if he was successful in acquiring a diploma abroad.

This difficulty presupposes his acceptance by a foreign medical school. In many cases, the criteria for admission are so high that he will not be accepted for study abroad if he was not accepted in the United States. Some foreign medical schools accept students with below-average qualifications and give them a chance to prove themselves. However, the scholastic standards at these schools are still high, and a large percentage of the class fails at each examination. Schools that graduate poorly qualified students do not produce doctors capable of obtaining United States certification.

Applying to a Foreign Medical School

The World Health Organization publishes a directory containing information about foreign medical schools, admission requirements, tuition, fees, and descriptions of the curriculum. This publication, *The World Directory of Medical Schools,* can be obtained for $6.75 per copy from: United Nations, Sales Section, Room

1059, New York, New York 10017, or from: Columbia University Press, International Documents Service, 2960 Broadway, New York, New York 10027.

Many consular offices will have descriptive materials and application forms for medical schools in their countries.

In many European countries, the number of seats available in medical schools to applicants from the United States is limited. Language is another barrier that should be of prime consideration. Unless you are fluent in the language of instruction, your difficulties in medical school will be multiplied as you try to absorb the course material. You should apply only in those countries whose language you have completely mastered. Some schools require foreign applicants to demonstrate language proficiency before their applications will be considered. Since most of the teaching in medical school is by means of lectures and examinations are usually oral, you will be overwhelmed if you have not mastered the language.

Many foreign schools request the MCAT scores of American applicants, in addition to their college transcripts. Medical education abroad often begins at an earlier level than in the United States. The average length of foreign medical education is about five years. The transfer of foreign credits to American medical schools is difficult, and years of study may be lost because of differences in the educational systems. Less than half of the medical schools in the United States are willing to consider students who transfer from foreign schools, even when they are well-qualified.[1]

If you plan to enroll in a foreign medical school, you first should consult the board of medical examiners of the state in which you plan to practice. Request the state's regulations regarding graduates of foreign medical schools and find out whether or not the school you are considering is acceptable to qualify you for licensure in that state. Although the American Medical Association recognizes as eligible for internship and residency a graduate of any foreign medical school if he has been certified by the Educational Council for Foreign Medical Graduates, some states have their own lists of approved schools and will license only graduates of those schools.[2] Additional information may be obtained from the American Medical Association, 535 North Dearborn Street, Chicago, Illinois 60610.

The Association of American Medical Colleges has prepared the following policy statement on United States requirements for foreign medical graduates:

United States students who graduate from foreign medical schools and wish to practice in this country must pass an examination given by the Educational Council for Foreign Medical Graduates (ECFMG), and they must satisfy the licensure requirements of the states in which they wish to practice.

ECFMG examination: The ECFMG examination consists of 360 questions of the multiple-choice type that are selected from a large pool of questions, used previously in . . . examinations of the National Board of Medical Examiners . . . this examination is given twice a year in centers all over the world and must be passed before a graduate of a foreign medical school, even though he is a United States citizen, can accept an internship or residency appointment in the United States. Furthermore, 40 states require ECFMG certification as a prerequisite for admission to their licensure examinations. In order to pass the ECFMG examination, a student must attain the same minimum score required of a graduate of a United States school.[3]

The Association of American Medical Colleges has prepared a reprint entitled *Information for United States Students who are Considering Earning a Medical Degree Abroad,* which can be obtained by writing to the association at 2530 Ridge Avenue, Evanston, Illinois 60201.

Additional information may be obtained from:

Educational Council for Foreign Medical Graduates
3930 Chestnut Street
Philadelphia, Pennsylvania 19104

The *Journal of the American Medical Association* publishes two special issues each year that should be read by the student contemplating foreign study. The state board number, in June, and the education number in November carry up-to-date information on this topic.

U.S. Internship and Residency for Foreign Medical Graduates

The National Internship Matching Program is available to, and is recommended for, graduates of foreign medical schools. Many hospitals use this plan exclusively in the selection of their interns.

The AMA recognizes as eligible for internship and residency training any foreign graduate who has been certified by ECFMG.

Internship should not be taken, either in the United States or abroad, until the student has obtained his M.D. and holds the ECFMG certificate. Earlier internship will not be recognized in the United States, even when credit for it has been granted by the student's foreign medical school.

U.S. Licensure of Foreign Medical Graduates

A graduate of a foreign medical school should be aware of the many and diverse regulations for obtaining a license to practice medicine in the various states.

To save time, money, and aggravation, the student should find out about the particular regulations of the state in which he wishes to practice during his years of preparation. Unless the student has complied with all the regulations, he may have great difficulty in obtaining an American license.

"To penetrate into the mysteries surrounding the licensing of foreign graduates requires the perspicacity of the art dealer, the nimbleness of the stock market speculator, and the doggedness of the bill collector. I know. I am a foreign medical graduate myself, but one of the American variety." [4]

Dr. Klaus Feuchtwanger has vivid memories of the lengthy bureaucratic ritual to which he was subjected in order to obtain his medical license after returning to America with an M.D. obtained in Switzerland. The story of Dr. Feuchtwanger and his family is a most unusual one and will serve to illustrate some needed improvements in our treatment of qualified physicians educated in foreign countries.

In considering applicants for licensure, state boards must, of course, exercise reasonable caution combined with a realistic evaluation of academic ability and professional skill. Instead, some of them tend to regard foreign medical graduates as a strange, "heterogeneous, unfortunate conglomeration of people, comprising students from somewhat off-center, at least medically, places," Dr. Feuchtwanger states.

His tongue-in-cheek description continues:

"The Doctor of Medicine licensed to practice in an exotic state such as, let us say, Michigan, is definitely an impostor and liable to severe penalties should he ever attempt to practice in the sovereign state of New York without first having submitted to the quite picturesque rules of the New York State Division of Professional Licensing." [5]

Since such attitudes of suspicion do exist in many states, notably New York, let the student beware!

Dr. Feuchtwanger and his wife, Dr. Rose-Andree Feuchtwanger, decided to enter medicine after eighteen years of marriage. They were then in their mid-forties, and upon application to several American medical schools they discovered that the opportunity to study medicine was closed to them in this country.

The Feuchtwangers were naturalized citizens of the United States who had resided in this country since 1939. Dr. Klaus was the owner and manager of a successful plastic products factory on Long Island, where the family lived. It was through the factory that the Feuchtwangers first became interested in psychiatry, because some of the workers had been patients at a nearby state hospital.

"Their adjustment or maladjustment intrigued me. These observations over a period of time condensed to a desire to study medicine and become a psychiatrist," Dr. Klaus says.

Dr. Rose-Andree admits that she had never really considered medicine as a career, although "I was always interested in people and their psychology." She had studied for one year at the Sorbonne in Paris before the couple came to the United States, and had planned to major in languages.

The Feuchtwangers took their premedical subjects, which they passed with top grades, and decided to make the break from their established, comfortable way of life.

"This was it," Dr. Klaus remembers. "I sold my factory and persuaded my wife to study medicine with me. For good measure, our daughter Michele, although a native-born citizen of the United States, enrolled with us at the University of Bern."

Once her husband had made his decision, Dr. Rose-Andree decided that she would share in the venture wholeheartedly. "I could not have had the courage or ambition to do it alone. But we always work together, so it seemed natural. We decided to go all the way." [6]

Dr. Klaus obtained his M.D., graduating at the top of his class, from the University of Bern in Switzerland. Since his wife was one year behind him in school, he obtained his ECFMG certificate and took an internship at a Swiss state hospital while she finished her senior year.

"My wife also took her internship in Switzerland, however, as

we both feel the Swiss training is superior to that of the United
States. It is a fallacy that American medicine is superior to the
entire world. Many countries of Europe are way ahead of America,
and we here in the United States do not wish to acknowledge this,"
Dr. Klaus explains.[7]

Dr. Rose-Andree had planned to specialize in internal medicine
but became intrigued with psychiatry because of her husband's intense interest in the field. "I thought it would not do me any harm
to work in psychiatry for one year. Once exposed, I took such a
liking to it that I couldn't do anything else now. In psychiatry, you
can see the whole patient."

The Feuchtwangers returned to their home on Long Island and
took positions as resident psychiatrists in the same state hospital
where some of their former employees had been patients. Their
daughter Michele, who had married a fellow medical student, remained behind, and she and her husband now live and practice in
Switzerland.

The long odyssey to obtain U.S. licensing now began. Dr. Klaus
believes that current methods of licensure in America need a lot of
overhauling and that uniform national standards should be established. "The idea of fifty little individual boards setting up fifty
different sets of standards in today's world of rapid communica-
tions is absurd."

The greatest difficulty the Feuchtwangers encountered was acceptance of their Swiss internships in the state of New York. At
one point, Dr. Klaus actually considered repeating his internship
(although he was already licensed in other states) in order to acquire a license to practice in New York. His training was so superior
that two federal hospitals told him there would be nothing he could
learn during an additional internship, in view of his extensive experience. By this time, he had completed his residency and held positions as senior psychiatrist and supervising psychiatrist in New
York State hospitals.

Dr. Klaus believes he has been more fortunate than many other
well-qualified physicians who spend years trying to acquire licenses
to practice in New York and some of the other states that "always
find something" as grounds for denial to anyone who is not a native
North American. With solid credentials plus years of perseverance
in cutting through the red tape, both of the Feuchtwangers finally
succeeded in amassing "such diverse trophies as a state board diploma of the Federal Republic of (Western) Germany, an M.D.

diploma from a Swiss University, state licenses (after written examinations) of New York and Georgia, and state licenses (by endorsement) of both Ohio and Michigan." [8]

Dr. Klaus is now director of the Steuben County Mental Health Service and has a private practice in upstate New York. Dr. Rose-Andree is a staff psychiatrist at Willard State Hospital in Steuben County, where they now reside.

Dr. Klaus believes he is as patriotic as the next man, but says that the United States does itself no good by policies of keeping out "foreigners" (including physicians from other states) and by maintaining that everything in America is automatically superior to anything elsewhere.

Curiously enough, a former president of the Federation of State Medical Boards of the United States admits that there is a continuing need for foreign medical graduates in our hospitals. If all states were to bar foreign medical graduates, he says, "the profession would soon become so inbred that the tenuous claim that the United States has the best medical care in the world would have no basis at all." [9]

Dr. Klaus believes strongly that "foreign medical graduates"—a term that is meaningless as an indicator of achievement in medicine —should be evaluated more realistically. It is a myth that American medicine is basically different from German, French, Swiss, English, or Italian medicine, and young people entering the profession in this age of international communication know it. There is such a great interchange of ideas, speakers, professors, programs, and textbooks among the western nations that the concept of "American medicine" is as unrealistic as that of "American physics" or "American chemistry."

The current acute shortage of seats available to qualified medical school applicants is one factor that contributes to the necessity for many students to pursue medical educations abroad. Also, students whose parents work overseas with American companies, or who have fathers in the military service, often find it more advantageous to study close to their current family residence.

It is outdated and provincial to regard with suspicion anyone who has not been educated on native soil.

"A medical student who obtains high marks in any western country is usually better versed in all branches of medicine than one who just passes," Dr. Klaus points out. Proficiency in medical matters may be lacking in graduates of American medical schools just the same as in graduates of schools in other western countries. In the case of such highly qualified applicants as the Feuchtwangers, rejection because of the single factor of age prompted them to turn to a country where they could be accepted into medical , school.

Dr. Klaus summarizes his hopes for future international cooperation and greater reciprocity among countries that share similar standards in medical education:

> If any American desiring to study medicine could be admitted to an American medical school, the need to go abroad would no longer exist. As long as sufficient facilities for medical training are unavailable—in spite of continuous need for more medical graduates—the American physician and the American taxpayer should be happy that some students are allowed to enroll in excellent foreign medical schools that are supported by foreign taxpayers. The American student abroad may bring home medical knowledge and medical skills equal, inferior, or superior to those of graduates from American medical schools; their respective achievements will be due not to the standards of their schools but to the personal endowment, perseverance, character, and intelligence of the individual student.
>
> And thus we may still the ghost of that ill-conceived monster, the "foreign medical graduate." [10]

Foreign Study Programs for Students of American Medical Schools

Students who desire to study abroad for the social and cultural experience would do well to consider taking their M.D. and internship in the United States, at the same time taking advantage of the many opportunities offered by U.S. medical schools to participate in special programs of study, clerkship, and directed research in all parts of the world. Fellowships are often available, particularly during the summer months, to pursue such interests. The honors program at the new Milton S. Hershey Medical Center of Pennsylvania State University, for instance, allows superior students to spend an elective period during their clinical years at a village medical facility in a developing country. More and more medical schools are including such international electives in their curricula.

The Public Health Service of the Department of Health, Education and Welfare grants fellowships for study abroad. For example, a fourth-year medical student at New York Medical College was recently granted a two-month fellowship for study in Yugoslavia by the Social and Rehabilitation Service of the PHS. Religious organizations also provide grants and travel expenses to eligible students. The Methodist Board of Missions has sent a senior medical student throughout Southeast Asia for observation and evaluation of medical installations. Medical missionary opportunities will be described later in this chapter.

Opportunities to Practice Medicine Abroad

Persons who have received their M.D.s and completed the required internships are eligible for a large variety of overseas opportunities for young physicians.

The Public Health Service cooperates with international health agencies, governmental and nongovernmental, and provides advice and assistance to countries throughout the world. The PHS is this country's official technical liaison with the World Health Organization (WHO), the directing and coordinating authority for all international health affairs. In the public health field, WHO assists countries in the development of such services as public health administration, nutrition, mental health, maternal and child health, nursing, health education, and social and occupational health.

WHO has granted thousands of fellowships to health workers throughout the world for the study of modern methods of combating disease. The staff of WHO numbers about three thousand, located at its Geneva, Switzerland, headquarters, at WHO regional offices, and on field assignments in 117 member countries. In the Americas, the regional office of WHO is: The Pan American Sanitary Bureau, Washington, D.C.

The Public Health Service offers opportunities for enriching medical service abroad at every level: student, physician, and paramedical. Unfortunately, the printed information of the PHS is vague and general. If your medical school will assist you in inquiring, or if you can talk in person with a visiting recruiting officer of the PHS, you will obtain more satisfactory information. If personal contact is not possible, write to the Public Health Service, U. S. Department of Health, Education, and Welfare, Washington, D.C. 20525. Indicate your individual career interests in your letter, and write back for a personal answer if the brochures do not provide the information you require. Persistence counts! Although the PHS is actively recruiting all types of medical personnel, the wheels of the bureaucratic system grind slowly. During the past year, the administrative structure of the PHS has undergone a tremendous change, with the names of many divisions being changed and information material revised. As a result, answers to correspondence take weeks, and sometimes months.

The Peace Corps. The Peace Corps employs doctors for salaried staff assignments overseas. The staff physician serves as general medical officer responsible for the physical and mental health of Peace Corps volunteers abroad, who average twenty-three years of age. The doctors have the option of working in local projects during their spare time.

Queries for information on this challenging opportunity should be made well in advance of the date on which you plan to file your application. The current Peace Corps recruiting brochure, which can be obtained from placement offices at most colleges, is a public relations piece that contains little specific information. The best bet is to secure information in person when a Peace Corps recruiter visits your campus or community.

Write to the Recruiting Office of Medical Programs, Peace Corps, Washington, D. C. 20525, for the booklet, *An Adventure in Medicine,* which details the responsibilities, experiences, qualifications, and projects of Peace Corps physicians. Questions on specific points of personal interest also should be directed to this office. The Peace Corps is actively recruiting female physicians and is eager to have them, but the necessary information is not readily available in many localities.

In addition to the salaried staff physicians whose primary job is taking care of the volunteers, the Peace Corps accepts doctors as volunteers. Like all corpsmen, these doctors receive a small living allowance and devote their time to working with the people of the country in which they are serving. At present the greatest need, however, is for staff physicians, because of the recent elimination of draft exemptions for Public Health Service doctors serving with the Peace Corps. The Military Service Act of 1967 stipulates that these physicians can no longer satisfy their military obligations by serving two years with the Peace Corps, and this stipulation has reduced greatly the corps' major source of staff physicians.

The Peace Corps therefore has turned to the entire American medical community to recruit physicians to care for the fourteen thousand volunteers serving in fifty-eight countries around the world. Today, there are about 140 staff physicians overseas. The physician is usually based in the foreign country's capital city or in a large provincial city, and is responsible for the clinical and preventive medical care of the volunteers in that country. He keeps their immunizations up to date, makes frequent visits to their working sites, and gives them any emotional support they may need while adjusting to their new circumstances. The staff physician also gives the volunteers lessons in health practices. "Doctors in the Peace Corps find that in some ways taking care of volunteers comes close to fulfilling the role that most physicians desire: the role of treating the whole person." [11]

To qualify for a Peace Corps assignment, a physician must be willing to serve two to three years overseas; must have completed one year's internship and be licensed to practice medicine in one of the fifty states or the equivalent; must be a United States citizen (spouse as well); and must not have served in any capacity with a government or military intelligence agency.

Peace Corps physicians' salaries start at $11,500 and range upward, depending on experience, training, and previous earnings. Annual leave arrangements are generous, and most American holidays and often the national holidays of the country of assignment are observed. Educational allowances are provided if the physician has children in elementary or secondary school. The Peace Corps ships household items to the country of assignment and pays for the storage of possessions left in the United States. The corps also provides housing, furniture, utilities, and transportation for physicians who are heads of households. [12] The Peace Corps provides medical supplies and a modest medical library.

The following special rules apply to the married female physician with a family:

> If the wife continues to be a dependent of the husband, he (not being her dependent) would be required to pay his own and the children's transportation overseas, though the wife's would be paid by the Peace Corps. For the same reason, she would not be allowed the same housing allowance overseas as physicians who are heads of households.
>
> If, on the other hand, the wife contributes more than 51% of the amount needed to support the husband, he can then be considered her dependent and entitled to both housing and his transportation overseas. [13]

Each Peace Corps physician (and spouse) attends a four-to-six-week orientation session in Washington prior to taking an overseas post. The Peace Corps also provides its doctors with language training where applicable.

During the orientation period, the doctor studies an extensive report on the medical conditions in his assigned country. The report details prevalent local diseases and disease vectors, describes the hospitals and clinics, and evaluates the adequacy of local medical practice. Upon arrival in the assigned country, the staff physician immediately assumes the care of the volunteers. He also meets with as many local physicians and visits as many hospitals and clinics as possible. A large part of the doctor's work consists of directing preventive medical programs carried out by volunteers, programs ranging from family planning to large-scale immunization. As one doctor working in Nigeria put it: "It is the first time that we don't have specialists and sophisticated equipment with which to make diagnoses. We have to depend upon our innate abilities as physicians. There are few experiences in the United States to compare to this."

Many woman physicians serve with the Peace Corps, and one of them described her assignment as a "natural profession for women" because the country in which she was working (Thailand) had such a high percentage—almost 50 percent—of women doctors.

Every effort is made to assign doctors to the countries they request. However, the needs of the Peace Corps change constantly, and it is these needs that determine the country of assignment. To prevent disappointment, the corps asks that physicians be prepared to accept assignments anywhere.

Private Programs and Foundations. There are many opportunities to practice medicine abroad, either for limited assignments—ranging from as little as one month to two years—or, as in the case of medical missionaries, for a lifetime. Doctors who serve in underdeveloped countries usually head teams of trained paramedical assistants. In the developed western countries, notably in Europe, medical fellowships are available for advanced study in various fields. Teaching appointments for physicians are another possibility for temporary assignment and cultural enrichment. Many foundations provide special grants to help strengthen the training of medical and nursing students, interns, and physicians in areas of acute medical scarcity.

An illustration of the variety of opportunities for service to others and for expansion of one's own experience and interests exists in MEDICO. Now affiliated with CARE, Inc., MEDICO was founded in 1958 by Dr. Peter D. Comanduras and the late Dr. Thomas A. Dooley to give developing countries the benefit of modern United States and Canadian medical practice. Its privately supported program is nongovernmental and nonsectarian. CARE maintains missions in thirty-five countries overseas to carry on its extensive relief work in selected areas of Asia, the Middle East, Africa, and Latin America. As many as sixty-five MEDICO doctors, nurses, and medical technologists are in residence overseas at any one time as members of long-term medical teams or as short-term volunteers.

At the invitation of host governments and in cooperation with local medical groups, MEDICO teams assist in meeting local health needs and training their counterparts abroad. Training of local medical staff is a priority goal; the program seeks to benefit the country in which the mission is established by training enough local personnel to carry on when the CARE-MEDICO team leaves. It is in neglected areas of the globe, where medical and scientific methods are deficient, that MEDICO intends to concentrate its activities.[14] A primary purpose of the program is to send American doctors to aid in organizing regional medical services and to practice medicine on the village level. Host governments are asked to underwrite the cost of living quarters, meals, local transportation, and necessary administration for MEDICO teams.

Rather than foster dependence on outside help, MEDICO hopes to raise the health standards of underdeveloped countries and bring the people to self-sufficiency in providing health care to their own. In Malaysia, two missions recently were declared "completed": the neurological unit founded in 1963 at Kuala Lumpur General Hospital was turned over to the host government; and the team at Kuala Lipis district hospital (founded by Dr. Thomas Dooley shortly before his death) was reduced, in preparation for closeout in 1968.[15]

Currently, MEDICO is active in three major fields: (1) long-term medical teams in Afghanistan, Algeria, the Dominican Republic, Honduras, Malaysia, and Tunisia; (2) short-term treatment and training programs by volunteer visiting specialists in Afghanistan, the Dominican Republic, Honduras, Malaysia, Tunisia, Vietnam, and occasionally other countries; (3) the International Eye

Foundation, which, through the Eye Bank, serves as a clearing-house for surplus corneas donated in the United States and Canada, flying them to fifty countries where transplant surgery can be done. The foundation sponsors an exchange of foreign and American ophthalmologists to further the spread of advanced eye surgery techniques and treatments. Continuing programs exist in Algeria, Jordan, and El Salvador, with plans for additional services in Tunisia, Liberia, and Honduras.

MEDICO personnel function either as members of long-term MEDICO teams or as short-term volunteer specialists.

Long-term MEDICO teams comprise certified and/or licensed physicians, nurses, and medical technicians with at least one year of postgraduate professional experience who have had a significant part of their training in North America. Team members serve overseas for two years, receiving substantial pay and living allowances. The sustained team programs support the work of local medical personnel.

Applicants for the long-term teams are required to undertake two-year assignments. Prior to an applicant's acceptance for service, a personal interview is required at CARE headquarters in New York. Knowledge of a second language, such as French or Spanish, is highly desirable.

Physicians receive salaries of $300 or $350 per month, plus a specific country subsistence allowance paid in the local currency. A team captain earns an additional $50 per month for his extra job responsibilities. Most doctors, nurses, and technicians serving with MEDICO have found it possible to save substantial amounts of their salaries. Personnel receive comprehensive insurance coverage, dental care, vacations every six months, and daily allowances for the physician (and his wife). Housing is provided by MEDICO or the host country. Air travel between the place of hire and the overseas post of assignment is provided for the physician, his spouse, and two children.

Augmenting the work of the MEDICO teams are the short-term volunteer specialists—internists, surgeons, and other specialists in all areas of medicine, who come from all parts of the United States and Canada. They spend a month each in program areas on a rotation basis, paying their own air fare and living expenses. Supplied by MEDICO and local sources with medicine and equipment, they teach and practice their disciplines. The orthopedics overseas division alone has furnished about one-third of the 650 specialists who have served in the last eight years.[16] This is a mission for established medical specialists who wish to broaden their professional background through experience with a variety of clinical patients and to contribute to a program that appeals to their idealism and concern for humanity.

Qualified medical and nursing teachers go abroad with MEDICO for varying lengths of time, visiting local schools on a lectureship basis.

The aim in detailing these aspects of MEDICO has been to acquaint you with the way in which such overseas programs function and to instill in young physicians the desire to share their knowledge with those less fortunate throughout the world, even if for only one month out of a lifetime. "Medical diplomacy" is one of the most effective means of showing—through work and involvement rather than talk—that Americans do care about other people in the world and are aware of the importance of international contacts on a personal, one-to-one level.

Further details on MEDICO can be obtained by writing to:

MEDICO, a Service of CARE
660 First Avenue
New York, New York 10016

Other foundations providing opportunities for service similar to MEDICO are: Thomas A. Dooley Foundation, 442 Post Street, San Francisco, California 94100; Laymen's Overseas Service, 321 Mississippi Street, Jackson, Mississippi 39201; Medical Operations Project Hope, People-to-People Foundation, 2233 Wisconsin Avenue, N.W., Washington, D. C. 20007.

Medical Mission Work. Medical mission work is carried on through the auspices of most major religious bodies. Mission associations sponsor installations throughout the world, often providing fellowships for short-term assignments to medical students and physicians. Further details can be obtained through your church. Some of the religious faiths and organizations that sponsor such programs are: the Roman Catholic, Episcopalian, Lutheran, Methodist, and Presbyterian Churches; also the Christian Medical Society, 1122 Westgate, Oak Park, Illinois 60311, and the World Brotherhood Exchange, Thousand Oaks, California 91360.

Notes to Chapter Eleven

1. *Medical School Admission Requirements, 1968–69,* Association of American Colleges, 1968. Appendix B. Reprinted by permission.
2. *Ibid.*
3. *Ibid.*
4. Klaus Feuchtwanger, M.D., "Of State Boards and Men," *Medical Opinion & Review,* Vol. III, No. 11, November, 1967.
5. *Ibid.*
6. Telephone interviews with Drs. Klaus and Rose-Andree Feuchtwanger, August 25 and 26, 1968.
7. *Ibid.*
8. Feuchtwanger, *op. cit.*
9. *Ibid.*
10. *Ibid.*
11. *An Adventure in Medicine:—The Peace Corps Staff Physician,* Peace Corps, Washington D.C., 1968.
12. Personal communication from Mrs. Doris A. Pointer, Administrative Assistant/Recruiting, Office of Medical Programs, Peace Corps, Washington, D.C., October 24, 1968.
13. *Ibid.*
14. *MEDICO, A Service of CARE,* New York, 1966.
15. Twenty-first Annual Report of CARE, Inc., New York, 1967.
16. *MEDICO, A Service of CARE.*

Chapter Twelve

INTERNSHIP

Now you are "Doctor." With a brand new M.D. and only one more year of required training before obtaining your license to practice, many choices are available. By the time a student reaches his senior year in medical school, he should have made the decision whether to enter general practice or to specialize. This will influence the type of internship for which he applies.

Choice of Internship

"Two types of internships are approved by the Council on Medical Education. They are:

"Rotating: . . . includes 12 to 24 months in two or more clinical services. At least four months must be in internal medicine. In a 12-month internship the remaining time may be divided between the surgical, pediatric, obstetrics-gynecology services, or major emphasis may be placed on a specific service for four to eight months. The great majority of physicians currently serve in rotating internships.

"Straight: In this type of internship, training is concentrated on a single medical, surgical, pediatric, obstetric-gynecology, or pathology service." [1]

Due to the greater emphasis on specialization, the current trend is toward straight internship. This type of training best meets the requirements of the majority of today's physicians.

"So many people are specializing today, it is becoming harder to find a university-type hospital that still carries the regular rotation program now," one dean states. "Our hospital has no rotating internships any more. Some of the big community hospitals carry them, and the military has them. Our interns take a straight internship with a major of six months in a particular service and electives thereafter."

When you apply for internship, you should consider the types of internships offered, the quality and emphasis placed on particular services, and the size and nature of the hospital and the community it serves.

Each year, almost one out of four available internships remains vacant. Of the 13,761 internships offered in September, 1967, only 10,419 were filled. Of this number, 2,913 were graduates of foreign medical schools.[2] We are not graduating nearly enough physicians to fill the demand. For the first time in his medical career, the student will find himself sought after and able to do some of the choosing. How wisely you choose will determine the course of your career for the rest of your professional life.

For the first time, also, the young physician begins to earn instead of spend. He no longer has to pay tuition, but receives a stipend, or annual salary, during the year of internship. In hospitals affiliated with medical schools, the average annual salary paid interns in 1968 was $4,139; it was $4,521 in hospitals not affiliated with medical schools. In general, stipends are highest in military training programs and lowest in hospitals affiliated with medical schools.[3] Specific information can be obtained from the *Directory of Approved Internships and Residencies,* published by the American Medical Association, 535 North Dearborn Street, Chicago, Illinois 60610.

Most institutions offer some or all of the following fringe benefits to their interns: housing, meal tickets, laundry service, insurance, and various other items that alleviate basic living expenses.

The internship usually lasts one, or sometimes two, years:

"The specialty boards have some specific requirements with respect to internship. Occasionally, two years of internship are necessary, but the one-year internship is usual, extending for 12 calendar months beginning on the first of July each year." [4]

Application for Internship

Medical students apply for internships during the fall of their senior year. Each individual usually applies to four or five hospitals. Many hospitals require personal interviews, and most students like to see the hospitals they are considering. Visits are made whenever possible, usually during the summer after the junior year. Some hospitals designate field agents in different localities—physicians known to the hospital administration who live in distant geographical areas. The field agent conducts personal interviews with students who desire an internship at the hospital he is representing but who cannot afford the trip to the hospital.

Most medical schools subscribe to the National Intern Matching Program. Participating students enroll with the program at the end of their junior year. The students can apply to as many hospitals as they wish. They submit individual applications to the hospitals of their choice, giving a copy of each application to their dean. Each participating hospital evaluates the applications it receives, lists them in order of preference, and often interviews the applicants personally. However, in keeping with the spirit of the plan, the hospital may not ask the student whether this is his number-one choice, nor may the student ask the hospital for his rating.

The student then lists the hospitals to which he has applied in the order of his preference. All the hospital and student preference lists are run through the organization's computer at Evanston, Illinois, and the student is assigned to the hospital highest on his list that has also selected him. Before the results are published, each student is sent a copy of his list for a double check, because each internship assignment that comes out of the computer is a contract.

As one dean described it: "The matching plan sends the results to all schools at the same time, on the same day, even taking into consideration the differences in the time zones. You can just watch the tension build as the day approaches. Every senior student is in a class meeting at the same time all over the country, opening the envelope to find out where he or she is going."

Further information on the program can be obtained by writing to: National Intern Matching Program, Attention: Executive Secretary, 2530 Ridge Avenue, Evanston, Illinois 60201.

Duties of the Intern

The intern is a member of the ward team under the direction of a faculty member and the resident staff. He is still in a learning situation, but carries much more responsibility than he did as a student. This gradual, step-by-step increase in responsibility is designed to augment the physician's versatility of experience with all types of patients suffering from all kinds of diseases. Part of the intern's training is duty in the hospital's emergency room and the treatment of outpatients in its various clinics. In the clinics, each department has an attending physician available to answer questions. In some of the services and subspecialties, such as dermatology or ear-nose-throat, most of the teaching is done in the clinic.

Although an intern has most of his classroom learning behind him, interns do not exchange their books for stethoscopes. They continue to read and review, often studying several hours each day to retain the material already learned and to keep abreast of new material constantly being added through research and discovery. By now, studying is a habit, which will be continued throughout their professional years. As one intern remarked: "You never stop studying. There must be a new disease discovered every month."

Advice to the lovelorn from experienced physicians runs from "Wait until you complete your training" to "At least finish the preclinical years before marrying." There are good reasons for such advice. The clinical years are tougher physically, but the basic learning has been completed. Internship is a matter of adjusting to a schedule, including being on emergency call one or two nights a week, but the satisfaction of finally being a physician seems to be reward enough for most of those plunged into this busy year.

The unmarried female physician, or at least the nonmother, will find her internship a year of achievement as well as learning. Once she has learned how to manage her time, she will be too busy, too involved, to worry about minor conflicts and inconveniences. But what about the girl who married in medical school, whose family has been started, and who must now combine increased family responsibilities with the busiest year of a physician's life?

The Mother-Intern

Dr. Lenor Zies had no intention of getting married before she finished medical school. Growing up in a family that numbered eighteen physicians among her relatives, Lenor decided as a very young girl to enter medicine. "I was going to be a doctor, regardless . . ."

When the family emigrated from Cuba to the United States, Lenor was fifteen years old. She attended high school in this country, mastered the English language, and won scholarships to finance her way through college. She accelerated at the undergraduate level in order to save money, completing her degree in three years.

"In high school and college, I was not so happy; I had to adjust to a different way of life. I really became adjusted to American life when I started medical school," she says.

At the age of nineteen, the youngest in her class, Lenor entered medical school. Despite her age and the disadvantage of studying in her second language, this talented student finished number two in her class the first year. Her Latin beauty and refined, old-world upbringing did not go unnoticed by the men in her classes. She dated several of her fellow students. Then—

"In my sophomore year, I married a classmate. Academically, my second year was a catastrophe. I became pregnant immediately and was sick the rest of the year. My class standing dropped from 2 to 25. But I have gotten so much out of my marriage that I don't regret it at all. These last four years have been the best years of my life."

Lenor discussed her family needs with her department chairman, and was permitted to make up during the summer the work she would miss in her junior year when the baby arrived. This arrangement is quite feasible during the clinical years, and most medical school deans express a willingness to cooperate on an individual basis with their married students.

By graduation day, Lenor had earned back her high class standing. Both she and her husband, Peter, had their M.D.'s, and they had a healthy young son to share their joy.

The experience of the Zieses and other young couples who marry and raise families during medical school indicates that certain conditions consistently seem to contribute to the success of the marriage-medicine combination. The fundamental condition is knowing what the career requires and preparing for the demands that will be made by family and profession.

First, the couple must have a realistic financial plan. Both husband and wife can surmount individual financial difficulties through scholarships, loans, and in some cases part-time work. Marriage brings the additional requirement of establishing a household, and children necessitate the expense of child care.

"If you are married and have children, you must have the means to get help in the house," Lenor emphasizes. "I have a full-time girl. It is impossible to manage without constant help. I don't attempt to do any housecleaning—it is bad enough to do the laundry and shopping. If you try to do too much, then you are too tired to study. We have a girl live in six days a week."

The Zieses are paying for this arrangement on their own, with careful budgeting. They each earn $375 a month as take-home pay from their internships. About $150 per month of their earnings goes to child care.

Both Lenor and Peter went heavily into debt for tuition in their last years of medical school (Lenor estimates that she already owes $7,000 for her education), although Peter's family helped with the living expenses after they married. Lenor points out that medical students can't count too heavily on earning additional money while in school:

"I did do summer work, but couldn't earn much . . . just enough to buy books and my microscope. Before graduation, you are a highly educated person who can't do anything."

A willing family that is solidly behind the marriage and the career ambitions of their children is a great asset. Lenor admits that the final two years of medical school were quite a financial imposition on the families. Although both she and Peter worked whenever possible at part-time duties, the year of internship was the first time they were able to cover all their own expenses.

After internship, there will be three years of pediatric residency for Lenor, and seven years of residency in surgery for Peter, who must follow this up with military service. Although Lenor's ultimate ambition is academic medicine ("I love to teach bright kids. Teaching others, you learn."), she plans to practice as a pediatrician until Peter is established as a surgeon, a goal that is probably ten years away.

Adequate child care is a most important consideration for the young marrieds in medicine who want to begin their families before they are established professionally. Child care means more than just having the child watched. All of the mother-doctors interviewed stressed the importance of providing the child with a warm, loving mother figure whose first concern would be the child's welfare during the mother's absence. Libby Connor found hers in a grandmotherly neighbor; Mabel Gibby and Ruth Lawrence rely on baby-sitters who come into the home and primarily care for the children, with household work taking secondary importance; Lenor Zies credits her mother with supplying the loving care her baby needs and deserves while she is at the hospital.

"I am very close to my family and chose to intern in this city because my family is here," Lenor said. "My mother helps with the baby—she has helped so much by giving my son the loving and cuddling he needs. She comes by almost every day and takes him for an outing while the girl does the housework. I don't think my son has suffered from lack of affection."

Lenor arrives at the hospital each day between 7:15 and 7:30 A.M. and checks each of her patients to see if any new problems have developed. Although she does not go on duty until 8:00 A.M., she believes early arrival is necessary "to make a decent presentation at rounds." Every fourth night she is on emergency call, and she alternates with another pediatric intern for weekend duties. Peter's schedule is more rugged because he is taking a straight surgery internship. He is on duty for twenty-four hours, then off for twenty-four hours. "You give up an awful lot of your social life during this time," Lenor admits.

When Lenor returns from the hospital each day, she plays with the baby for two hours. After he is in bed for the night, she does her studying.

Lenor adds that Peter, Jr., understands the difference between his parents' work and their social activities.

"When he sees us dressed in our white uniforms, he just waves bye-bye and does not make a fuss. He accepts it. When we go to leave the house dressed in street clothes—that is a different story. He cries and wants to go with us."

The kind of man a woman doctor marries is the catalyst that makes all the other elements of the medicine-marriage mixture combine. His maturity, his sincerity in sharing his wife's goals and ambitions, his willingness to share her with the demands of her profession, and his security in his own capabilities will determine whether the couple's home life is smooth or abrasive.

Despite the denials of some women, the doctor-doctor marriage seems to be the most successful and mutually compatible.

Lenor states flatly: "I know of very few marriages to men other than doctors that have worked for woman physicians. My husband is going through the same thing I am, so he understands. When I am on call, he gets dinner. When I have been on call the previous night, he takes the baby out so I can sleep. When he is on call, I do these things. It is never a question of husband's duty or wife's duty —it is a mutual helping for whoever needs it at the time."

Lenor tells her unmarried friends in medicine not to get involved with men outside the field. She believes that most nondoctors cannot help but be jealous of the achievements of their wives, with the result that friction and competition enter the marriage. She is grateful that she does not have to cope with a husband who wants to go out all the time, or who needs her attention to bolster his ego.

The woman doctors interviewed who were married to men outside the medical profession emphasized that, for the marriage to be happy, it was important for the husband to be successful in his chosen field and satisfied with what he was doing. He must be sufficiently mature to be proud of his wife's achievement, rather than feel threatened by it.

The Zieses are expecting their second child, and the new baby will be born right in the middle of Lenor's year of internship. They planned to have the second child at this time in order that the two youngsters could be raised together. Lenor intends to work until just before the baby is born, as she did with her first. Then she will take her two weeks' vacation plus one additional week, which she will have to make up, and has arranged her internship schedule accordingly.

"I talked with my department chairman before I even became pregnant and told him honestly of my family plans. When I knew my due date, I then requested the senior resident to schedule me for an 'easy' service the month before and after my delivery. The hospital has been very accommodating, and I am not losing time on my training. As a result, you cannot call mine a typical internship. I began with my elective, but I will complete the full year's work on schedule."

Dr. Lenor Zies has demonstrated that by facing each situation honestly and planning realistically, medicine can be compatible with raising a young family. She made her decisions fully aware of what was required from her in each area of her responsibilities. A woman without a helpful, sympathetic husband and family, or with inadequate means to pay for help in the nursery and household during this time, would be well-advised to postpone starting her family until completing her training.

Has it all been worth it? Lenor considers the question pensively for a minute and then admits, "I am only twenty-three years old, and my really fun years have been spent studying. I know there are other things in life besides closing yourself in a book. We love music and art. Those dabbles you see around the room—they are my husband's." She gestures at some modern paintings on the wall of the cozy living room. She smiles confidently and adds, "I am happy with what I am doing. My philosophy is that if I have half a glass of something, it is half full, not half empty. This contentment with what you have in life I learned from my father as a little girl. I love medicine. I couldn't be happier."

Old and New Attitudes Toward Internship

The demands and difficulties of internship should not be minimized, but they can be faced and resolved. Many women are overly sensitive about accepting any modifications of training that would set them apart from their male peers. Interns as a group often accept the most rigorous schedules and working conditions as part of the "hazing" necessary for full "admission to the club." This attitude might explain the reluctance of interns, men and women, to complain about long working shifts or the traditional schedule—a "lockstep twenty-four hours on, twenty-four hours off," as one administrator described it.

Such acquiescence is false pride on the part of a mother who must cope with the realities of sick children, an occasional "no-show" baby-sitter, or some other domestic calamity. The best solution, of course, is a more understanding system of internship for both men and women. Men, too, require time off for illness or family crises. A climate of give-and-take, rather than of striving to prove who is the most superhuman in dedication, would lessen tensions throughout this demanding year.

New plans and programs designed to modify the inflexibility of postgraduate medical training are detailed and evaluated in Part III.

Notes to Chapter Twelve

1. *Horizons Unlimited,* American Medical Association, 1968. P. 48.
2. Personal communication from Hayden C. Nicholson, M.D., Director of Division of Medical Education, American Medical Association, September 19, 1968. Statistics published in *Journal of the American Medical Association,* November, 1968.
3. *Medical School Admission Requirements,* 1968–69, Association of American Medical Colleges, 1968. P. 45 and table 5.5. Reprinted by permission.
4. *Op. cit.* P. 43.

Chapter Thirteen

CHOICE OF SPECIALTY AND THE RESIDENCY

The General Practitioner

In private practice, the proportion of specialists has been increasing to the point where they outnumber general practitioners two to one among active M.D.'s. The American Academy of General Practice reports that less than 2 percent of all 1967 medical school graduates chose to enter general practice, and this is a field in which women can do very well. General practitioners, or "family physicians," treat the whole patient, not just the afflicted part. Their practice takes in patients of all ages, since they are doctors for all the members of a family.

As one young woman intern put it: "The nature of general practice appeals to me strongly. You get to treat the whole family. If the child is having trouble with his parents, you know them and can call them in."

If a group practice is possible, the woman general practitioner can arrange her office hours and emergency-call nights on a predictable schedule that will be manageable along with the demands of family life. For those who find variety stimulating, nothing can take the place of general practice. In addition to being a diagnostician, therapist, and counselor, the family physician practices preventive medicine, maintaining and promoting the health of entire families.

Family Medicine. New emphasis is being placed today on training physicians for the discipline of family medicine, or family practice. The family physician is a specialist in the continuity of health management, rather than just providing continuing treatment for a specific illness. The family physician is described as a "cross between the private practitioner and the public health doctor, with the primary interest centered on the basic sociological unit of our society, the family, instead of the individual." [1]

The concept of family medicine is not identical to that of general practice. The latter is disease-centered and implies episodic care. Family medicine is health-oriented and based on comprehensive care of the family. Besides practicing medicine, the family physician draws on the social sciences, psychology, and other disciplines in order to keep the entire family well.

In February, 1969, the Council on Medical Education of the American Medical Association and the Advisory Board for Medical Specialties approved the establishment of the new specialty of family medicine. Recognition of family practice as a specialty is expected to give it the status, privileges, and pay of the other specialties. As a consequence, it is hoped that increasing numbers of medical students will enter this specialty in both urban and rural areas. The establishment of family medicine as a specialty in its own right is also expected to restore entrée to hospital staffs for general practitioners, who in recent years have been shunned by many medical centers and teaching hospitals.

The education and residency requirements for family medicine are comparable to those of most other specialties, with three years of graduate work following four years of medical school. Physicians passing new certification board examinations will become diplomates in family medicine, with the same specialty rank and status as diplomates in the other specialties. Unlike the other specialties, however, the family practice board will require periodic recertification by examination.

Many medical schools recognize our nation's growing need for a constant supply of family physicians to provide the modern, complete health care that Americans demand, and are taking active steps to prepare more medical students for this role. Approximately 25 percent of the medical schools in the United States have programs in operation, or are planning them, in comprehensive family health care. Two schools, Harvard Medical School and the University of Miami (Florida) School of Medicine, have postgraduate fellowship programs to prepare physicians who have completed their training, or have been in practice, for academic careers in family medicine.[2]

The University of Miami's medical school has developed an elective in family medicine that is handled as a subspecialty of the Department of Medicine. Dr. Lynn Carmichael, director of the program, believes there is a distinct difference between general practice and family medicine. He defines family medicine as the branch of medical science that has as its responsibility the continuing health maintenance of the family. As an academic discipline, it has a distinct body of knowledge and is housed in the university. Others besides physicians are involved in the discipline. The general practice of medicine is directed toward the delivery of medical care and involves the episodic treatment of disease. The goal of family medicine is service, and there are cultural, political, and economic overtones.

Medical students, interns, residents, and fellows participate in the Miami program. The heart of the teaching and research activity is the supervised care of families in an ambulatory care facility. Over 250 families receive continuing and comprehensive health care in the Family Health Center. In addition to the clinical service, there are case presentations, conferences, and lectures for the participating students and physicians.

The objective of the undergraduate program, according to Dr. Carmichael, is to encourage the development of positive attitudes in students about comprehensive family care. No tests or grades are given, although an evaluation of each student is made. In the junior year, each student is assigned to a family and serves as its family physician under the close supervision of the program's staff. A full range of medical services is provided to the family, including periodic health evaluation for all family members, prenatal care, and attention during periods of illness. The service center of the program is the ambulatory facility, where the families are examined by appointment. The student assigned to a particular family is notified by mail or telephone of the appointment and is excused from his regular clerkship in order to be present. Home visits are a regular part of the care offered to the family, and are encouraged. A member of the staff must accompany the student on every home visit.

The families who receive care at the Family Health Center have been referred by private practitioners, community agencies, and other sources. Most of them are nonindigent and represent a wide distribution of social, economic, and cultural characteristics. An effort is made to select families that span three generations, preferably including an expectant mother, to give the students the experience of practicing throughout the age spectrum.

The program provides students with their only opportunity while in medical school to observe continuing health care of a family. They also attend regularly scheduled conferences and are welcome guests at other departmental meetings. Fellowship applications should be made during the summer between the student's third and fourth years. During the fourth year, the student may arrange to spend from one to four months in family medicine as a senior elective.

The graduate program at the University of Miami School of Medicine offers three years of training—one year of internship and two years of residency. Interns are encouraged to continue into residency, and to serve as family physicians for assigned families throughout their training. Interns, residents, and fellows work under the supervision of practicing family physicians and attend conferences, seminars, and discussion groups. Each resident is expected to conduct a research project in patient care (rather than clinical or basic research). Interns and residents also rotate through the various specialty services. The interns spend six months in internal medicine, four in pediatrics, and two in obs' .t-rics-gynecology.

Dr. Carmichael believes that the most innovative programs utilizing the special training of the family physician are the Neighborhood Health Centers developed by the Office of Economic Opportunity. He sees these centers as the forerunners of new family-oriented medical institutions, distinct from hospitals, that will provide comprehensive, continuing health care through their community-based physicians.

Another example of important new developments is the Department of Family and Community Medicine at the Hershey Medical Center of Pennsylvania State University College of Medicine. This new college of medicine, which enrolled its first class in 1967, stresses the concept of medical practice as an art with a scientific base: "Understanding of people, their backgrounds and reactions, is essential to provide optimal patient care." [3]

The college integrates the teaching of family and community medicine with the practice of selected family physicians in the community who are full-time faculty members. The physicians have full hospital admitting privileges and see their patients in offices in the college's Medical Sciences Building. During the first week of school, each student in the program is assigned a family to care for through the four years of medical school and, in so doing, to follow continuously the impact of disease on the family and the community.

Hershey Medical Center is an innovator in other areas as well, emphasizing the importance of individual study, small classes, and a high faculty-student ratio in an informal environment. Hershey also has an honors program that allows students to spend an elective period during the clinical years at a village medical facility in a developing country.

Appropriate Internship. Students who plan to enter general practice and whose medical schools do not have a family medicine program would be wise to seek out the hospitals offering internships affiliated with such a program, or take regular rotating internships. Of particular value is a hospital in a large metropolitan area with a wide variety of departmental outpatient clinics. Training at such a hospital provides the broadest possible base in treating ambulatory patients with the diseases that are frequently encountered in the offices of general practitioners.

Previously, evidence of competence in general practice was indicated by membership in the American Academy of General Practice, which required two years of graduate education approved by the academy and 150 hours of acceptable continuation study every three years.[4] Further particulars may be obtained from the Academy: Volker Boulevard at Brookside, Kansas City, Missouri 64112.

Physicians now in general practice may take the examination in family medicine upon completing three hundred hours of accredited postgraduate study in medicine. There is no clause in the qualifications for the new specialty that permits automatic certification. The American Academy of General Practice expects to change its name to the American Academy of Family Physicians as soon as the changeover to the new specialty becomes fully effective.

The Other Specialties

Today there are twenty major fields of medical specialization in addition to general practice that are recognized by the American Medical Association. Within some of these specialties are recognized fields of subspecialty. The certification of diplomates in the specialties (except for administrative medicine) and subspecialties is administered by nineteen examining and certifying boards that have been approved by the Council on Medical Education of the American Medical Association and the Advisory Board for Medical Specialties.[5]

The major medical specialties are listed below, with the length of the required residency in parentheses:

Administrative medicine deals with the administration of medicine in business, health programs, and hospitals.

Anesthesiology deals with the administration of various forms of anesthetic drugs necessary during surgical operations or diagnosis (two- and three-year residency programs).

Colon and rectal surgery deals with the diagnosis and treatment of disorders or diseases of the lower digestive tract (five years, three general surgery and two of specialization).

Dermatology deals with the diagnosis and treatment of diseases of the skin (three years).

Internal medicine deals with the diagnosis and nonsurgical treatment of diseases of the internal organs such as the heart, liver, and lungs (excluding obstetrics-gynecology); a specialist in internal medicine treats diseases of adults and is primarily a diagnostician (three years).

Neurological surgery deals with the diagnosis and surgical treatment of the brain, the spinal cord, and nerve disorders (four years).

Obstetrics and gynecology deals with the diagnosis and treatment of diseases of the female reproductive organs and with the care of women during and immediately following pregnancy (three years).

Ophthalmology deals with the diagnosis and treatment, including surgery, of diseases or defects of the eye (three years).

Orthopedic surgery deals with the diagnosis and medical or surgical treatment of diseases, fractures, and deformities of the bones and joints (four years, one of general surgery and three of specialization).

Otolaryngology deals with the diagnosis and treatment of diseases of the ear, nose, and throat (four years, one of general surgery and three of specialization).

Pathology is the study and interpretation of changes in organs, tissues, cells, and body chemistry (three or four years).

Pediatrics deals with the prevention, diagnosis, and treatment of children's diseases (two years).

Physical medicine and rehabilitation deals with the diagnosis of disease or injury in the various systems and areas of the body, treatment by means of physical procedures, and treatment and restoration of the convalescent and physically handicapped patient (three years).

Plastic surgery deals with corrective or reparative surgery to restore deformed or mutilated parts of the body or improve facial or body features (five years, three of general surgery and two of specialization).

Preventive medicine (public health) deals with the prevention of disease and promotion of health through epidemiological studies and public health measures (two years).

Psychiatry and neurology deals with the diagnosis and treatment of emotional disturbances, mental disorders, and organic diseases affecting the nervous system (three years).

Radiology deals with the diagnosis and treatment of disease through the use of radiant energy, including X rays, radium, and cobalt 60 (three years).

Surgery deals with the diagnosis and treatment of disease, injury, or deformity by manual or operative procedures (four years, or three years of general and two years of special training).

Thoracic surgery deals with the diagnosis and operative treatment of diseases of the chest, including those involving the heart, lungs, and large blood vessels within the chest (two years).

Urology deals with the diagnosis and treatment of diseases and disorders of the kidneys, bladder, ureters, urethra, and the male reproductive organs (four years).

The above descriptions of specialties were taken from *Horizons Unlimited,* published by the American Medical Association in 1968.

A total of thirty-four medical specialties and subspecialties, in addition to general practice, are recognized by the American Medical Association. Some of the subspecialties are aerospace medicine, allergy, anesthesiology, child psychiatry, cardiovascular disease, and occupational medicine.

Descriptions of the specialties, prepared by the American Specialty Boards, are available from the Association of American Medical Colleges. The association's publication, *Medical School Admission Requirements,* lists the American Specialty Boards and their addresses, and contains a summary table of specialty training requirements, including prerequisites.

The American Medical Association's publication, *Essentials of Approved Residencies,* also lists the specialty boards and their addresses, and states which boards certify physicians in the various subspecialties. The AMA stresses that physicians who take hospital residencies and anticipate certification by specialty board should communicate with the secretary of the appropriate board at the outset of the residency training to acquaint himself fully with all the requirements. This publication describes the general requirements for approved residency programs and the special requirements for residency training in each of the approved specialties. It also delineates the personal and medical qualifications expected of applicants to the resident staff.

Internal Medicine. In this highly specialized age, internal medicine has taken over so many of the functions of general practice that the internist is often confused with the general practitioner. However, the tongue-in-cheek description of the internist as "a doctor who specializes in general practice" is not entirely accurate. The internist, for example, does not practice obstetrics, pediatrics, or surgery, while the general practitioner often does. Internal medicine is restricted to the diagnosis and treatment of internal disorders of adults.

Preparation for this specialty includes a wide background in the basic sciences and the various branches of medicine. The internist must know his abilities and limitations well enough to recognize when he needs to call in another specialist. He should always be aware of the patient as a whole person, not as a conglomeration of isolated organs or structures.

The practice of internal medicine presents most of the same demands as are made on the family physician and can be handled in much the same manner by a woman who wishes to combine this specialty with marriage and raising a family. Group practice is one solution, or in a community with need the physician can devise ways in which to offer effective service and educate the community to accept the hours she has to offer.

Part-time work is readily available to the internist in many areas. Working in a clinic or teaching in a local hospital or medical school will keep her informed of the newest procedures in the field. Private industry and business offer a great variety of positions, ranging from a few hours a day to seasonal or temporary work. Colleges report more openings for woman internists than physicians to fill them. Insurance companies, schools, colleges, camps, businesses, and community clinics offer opportunities for practicing internal medicine under controlled conditions.

Surgery. One specialty that is not recommended for women who plan to marry and raise a family while continuing to train and practice is surgery. Dropping out of the profession temporarily would make one's techniques so obsolete as to be almost irreparable. Certain types of surgery encompassed within other specialties permit modified practice, but general surgery demands long hours. Women practicing general surgery usually advise other women to be very cautious when considering this field, and realistic about what will be required of them.

Surgery is one specialty where considerable prejudice exists toward women, and sometimes with reason. Competition is keen for the surgical residencies, and department heads usually prefer to select the most qualified male candidates rather than risk placing a woman in a position where even a temporary withdrawal would work a hardship on the department that depends on her constant ability to serve.

Surgery is a demand specialty, with long hours and considerable emergency duty. A woman with small children would find it most difficult to cope with such a schedule, unless she were employed by an agency such as the Veterans Administration and her hours on duty were guaranteed. The best time for children to arrive is between the residency and the entrance into surgical practice, as a mother could not adequately cope with a family during a full-time residency. Once the residency is behind her, a mother-surgeon could accept a position as a surgical assistant at a hospital. In this way, she could maintain her techniques until her family was grown enough for her to be away from them for the long hours necessary to handle a surgical practice.

Residency

The average annual stipend of a resident (1968 figures) is little more than that of an intern. The average salary for the first year of residency in hospitals affiliated with medical schools is $4,095; it is $4,557 in hospitals not affiliated with medical schools. There is, however, a wide salary range after the first year, and senior residents in some institutions earn as much as $9,000 to $11,500 per year.[6]

In addition to stipends, there are national loan programs and local loan funds to help with expenses during postgraduate training. Loans are usually administered by the hospital, the state, or the local medical association. Loan information will be available at the hospital where you plan to take your residency.

There are also special grants for various purposes, and some specialty boards provide funds for postgraduate training, either for general usage or special purposes.

Certain types of residency training are subsidized in order to encourage physicians to enter a needed specialty, or to keep a continuing supply of specialists flowing into a given institution. Examples of subsidized training are the career residency program of the Veterans Administration and the United States government's program to encourage general practitioners to obtain postgraduate training in psychiatry.

Organizations that are sources of nonrefundable aid and loans for interns and residents are described in Chapter Nine. Extended training programs with stipends for mother-physicians and retraining programs for mothers who have left the field are detailed in Part III.

The demand for residents in United States hospitals also far exceeds the supply, and the shortage is even more critical than in the case of interns. In September, 1967, 41,695 residencies were offered. Only 33,743 of these were filled; the rest remained vacant. Of the positions filled, 10,627 were by graduates of foreign medical schools. In other words, about 18,000 more residents are needed each year than this country has available.[7]

Mother-Residents

Many female medical students put off marriage and childbearing until after completion of their medical education, and frequently until after the demanding year of internship. Those who are going on to specialize, however, usually take a now-or-never attitude and begin their families at the beginning of the internship and residency. It is at this stage that the danger of dropping out is most severe and that modification of traditional schedules can be instigated most effectively. Pilot programs in extended residencies and their success to date are described in Part III.

As Carol Lopate summarizes it in her book, *Women in Medicine:* "One means of decreasing the possibility of withdrawal by woman residents involves a concession on the part of their department heads (as well as the American Specialty Boards) to a less demanding schedule. Such a concession, however, could in time make an important contribution to medical womanpower." [8]

"In the spring of 1967, the major specialty boards supplied information on their policies regarding part-time residencies for women with dependent children."

Specialty boards that accept part-time residencies are anesthesiology, dermatology, psychiatry-neurology, and public health. Those that will consider modifications occasionally, on an individual basis, are internal medicine, pediatrics, and radiology. Those that will not accept any training other than the traditional full-time residency are obstetrics-gynecology, ophthalmology, pathology, and general surgery. [9]

The rulings delineated by the specialty boards regarding the structure of the residency programs are quite broad. The chairman of the department of a particular service has considerable latitude in designing the program at his hospital and often can make special arrangements to suit the needs of a qualified woman physician who takes the initiative to request modified or extended scheduling in her training. Both interns and residents attest to the fact that many department chairmen are cooperative in this regard and help women to manage pregnancy, maternity leave, or attention to small children during their residencies.

The greatest obstacle to mother-doctors seems to be the attitude of both the hospital administration, and the staff and co-workers. The negative attitude of co-workers is particularly hard to bear— when a mother needs time off, she often is resented by her male colleagues simply because she is a woman, even though these same male residents often require time off to cope with family emergencies of their own. When extended or part-time residencies have the official approval of the hospital administration, such tensions are lessened. Also, a climate of cooperation eases the training modifications that are needed to help mother-physicians remain active in their profession and still acquire the lengthy postgraduate training they must have to pursue today's specialized medicine.

Notes to Chapter Thirteen

1. Lynn P. Carmichael, M.D., "Teaching Family Medicine," *Journal of the American Medical Association,* Vol. 191, No. 1, January 4, 1965.
2. Carmichael, "Developments in the U.S.A.," position paper delivered at conference on Training in Family Medicine, sponsored by Association of Canadian Medical Colleges and College of General Practice in Canada, May 14, 1968.
3. *Medical School Admission Requirements,* 1968–69, Association of American Medical Colleges, 1968. P. 204. Reprinted by permission.
4. *Op. cit.* P. 43, table 5.3.
5. *Horizons Unlimited,* American Medical Association, 1968. Pp. 49 and 50.
6. *Medical School Admission Requirements,* 1968–69. P. 45 and table 5.5. Reprinted by permission.
7. Personal communication from Hayden C. Nicholson, M.D., Director of Division of Medical Education, American Medical Association, September 19, 1968. Statistics published in *Journal of the American Medical Association,* November, 1968.
8. Carol Lopate, *Women in Medicine,* Johns Hopkins Press, 1968. Pp. 132, 133, and table 8–2.
9. *Ibid.*

PART III

WOMAN'S ROLE IN THE
NEW AGE OF MEDICINE

Chapter Fourteen

TAKE THE INITIATIVE

Women in medicine in the United States today function in a man's world. Even if all the proposed programs to introduce flexibility into medical education were put into immediate action—and the prospect of such an about-face is dim—it would be decades before the numbers of male and of female medical students approached equality. Women, therefore, must be prepared to take the initiative; they must seek out information and work for needed changes at every stage of their preparation for a career in medicine.

From the beginning of your high school education, never take "no," "I don't know," or "we don't have that" for an answer. High school and premedical counseling, particularly as it affects girls, has been criticized strongly by many of today's medical educators. High school counselors often try to discourage girls from attempting medical careers, unaware that a woman has the same opportunity for acceptance into medical school as a man—once she reaches the applicant pool. If your school advisers do not come up with specific answers, contact your local medical society for information regarding prerequisite course work and early preparation. Consult Part I of this book and follow every suggestion that may provide you with the information you need. Attend meetings in your community designed to acquaint students with the medical profession.

Do not be discouraged by warnings against opportunities for women in medicine. This book has provided many models of successful women who are enjoying satisfying careers along with marriage and motherhood. Every community has its own similar examples. Ask your medical society or family physician if there is a woman doctor who would be willing to meet with a group of interested students.

To qualify for medicine, you must acquire in high school a thorough groundwork in mathematics and the sciences. If any courses you require or want to take are not available in your school's curriculum, enroll for summer courses wherever they are offered. Investigate the possibility of advanced-placement courses at a local college or university. Many medical schools strongly recommend calculus before entering medical school, especially for students applying for the new accelerated curricula that combine medical education with the arts and sciences. You can take calculus in summer school at any accredited college before entering premedical study.

Dr. Mary I. Bunting, president of Radcliffe College, recommends that girls take advantage of every opportunity to work in jobs related to medicine, and to begin seeking such contact with the profession early—even in high school. Although many girls do not make the final decision to enter medicine until the end of their undergraduate college education, studies of Radcliffe undergraduates have revealed that most decisions *against* entering medicine were made during the freshman and sophomore years of college.[1]

Dr. Bunting believes that there are not enough good chances during the college years for students to discover or confirm an interest in medicine. "Many more opportunities for summer field experiences related to medicine as well as opportunities to take courses in the medical schools ought to be available—and before the end of the sophomore year," Dr. Bunting states.[2]

It is up to the individual to test her interest in the medical profession by asking for job information and taking advantage of student placement programs wherever they are offered. Many gifted students from high school science classes are offered the chance to work in laboratories during the summer and discover fields previously unknown to them that offer fascinating careers in medicine.

Once a woman is enrolled in medical school, she should attempt to be assigned a female adviser. As long as scheduling is designed by men for men and the ratio of woman students to the class total is low, a female physician who could be consulted on career planning throughout the years of medical school is invaluable to a woman student. Try to locate a sympathetic and concerned female faculty member (or members) and ask her to set aside a time for consultation during her regular office hours, or to participate in an occasional group seminar where the woman students could discuss problems of common interest.

The Association of American Medical Colleges is concerned about the doctor dropout rate and recommends an active effort to decrease the attrition among medical students. Intensive counseling programs are suggested to prevent students from leaving for non-academic reasons.[3] Many woman doctors who are now inactive have complained, in various surveys, that they were poorly prepared for the dual role of a woman doctor. By expressing your views on the importance of realistic preparation and the need for continuing guidance throughout medical education to your department chairmen, medical school deans, and members of the administration, you can work toward establishing effective counseling services at medical schools where none exist.

Extended residencies and flexible postgraduate training programs have been worked out at several institutions on an individual basis *when a woman took the initiative to make such an arrangement.* "These programs are given no publicity, nor are candidates sought for them," Dr. Ruth Lawrence pointed out in her report to the Macy Conference. "Indeed, no counseling is given a woman by most medical schools to encourage her to seek out a means of completing her training."

Many women doctors report cooperation from their department heads in arranging individual schedules to allow for a maternity leave or a short break from their education for family responsibilities. However, every girl should keep in mind that, in the majority of cases, medical schools and hospitals alike do not encourage this flexibility and do not advertise its availability.

"One hears of opportunities only by chance, and only by perseverance is one able to work out something for herself if she finds a sympathetic ear," says Dr. Lawrence.

In postgraduate training, "residencies, and to a lesser extent internships, are departmentally controlled and not institutionally controlled . . . there is nothing to prevent a service chief from introducing whatever flexibility is necessary." [4]

Should the need for a flexible schedule arise, consult your department chairman or guidance counselor if one is available. Many department heads have told Dr. Lawrence that they would consider working out special programs if anyone asked for them. Several medical school administrators expressed a similar willingness to this author when polled by a questionnaire. Many men in positions of authority are cooperative when confronted with a specific situation and asked for help. It is up to the women to make their needs known, to present their requests honestly, and to suggest realistic alternatives to the current rigid requirements. This is a far better option than enduring conflict, losing training time, or dropping out altogether.

Women who have completed their training and are in positions of authority can initiate new programs and ideas beneficial to medical education in general and to women in particular. They must make certain, however that any proposed innovation meets standards comparable to those of the regular program. Alterations should be made in time schedules, not in the quality or overall quantity of training. Established physicians can work to innovate and implement new programs that will enable more women to participate in medicine.

Dr. Helen Kaplan, who worked to establish the mother-residents program at New York Medical College (*see* Chapter 17), advises that a woman interested in establishing a similar program should design it herself.

"Our program can serve as a model, but the basic interest must come from the woman herself. First, she must feel secure in her own femininity; then she has to at least try and fail." You will never realize the potential of your ideas if you do not try. Dr. Kaplan adds that the women in her program admitted they would never have attempted such a venture on their own; yet now they are participating successfully in the pioneer residency.

Dr. Glen Leymaster, president and dean of the Woman's Medical College of Pennsylvania, sees two options for the woman who needs specialized, individualized training with extended time schedules. She must be prepared to go to a school where such a program is offered. Or, "if she is an energetic self-starter, she can do the same thing for herself. This takes a lot more initiative and self-confidence," Dr. Leymaster believes.

Dr. Leymaster points out that, even without the help of a medical school to work out a specialized program, there are retraining opportunities in hospitals and medical institutions in almost all parts of the country.

"With very little review time, a woman doctor could do enough useful work to secure herself a position someplace and then carry on with her professional rehabilitation. She should seek out a well-developed medical center in her area, preferably one with a medical school, and ask to be retrained while she contributes whatever she can."

"Professional advancement in the medical world is one area where those women who claim prejudice have the facts on their side," Carol Lopate states in her book, *Women in Medicine.*[5]

"Women do not advance in staff positions in the medical schools, hospitals, or other institutions at the same rate as men. Out of 1,047 department chairmen in 78 United States medical schools, only 13 are women; there are only 105 women with the rank of professor, as compared to 2,554 men. At the lower end of the academic ranks, however, women take up far more than their 6 percent of the total medical population: 770 women are instructors and 2,132 men hold the same rank; 104 women are senior instructors, while 263 senior instructors are men." [6]

Dr. Leymaster believes that women themselves may be responsible for such small ratios, and offers an explanation:

"I have sought qualified women for positions as department chairmen. After being interviewed, they tell me they do not want to be in the competitive position of a chairman. I feel the opportunity to progress into positions of leadership is related to interest and ability, and the women are often content to be in the number two position. It is a matter of whether or not a person will want to compete for this responsibility, and I find, personally, that the women do not."

The woman's mobility, her commitments to her home once it has been established, and her husband's job are other important factors. To attain a position of leadership, a woman must be prepared to move. It is unlikely that her husband will leave his job to accommodate his wife's desire to advance in her profession. Women with families often prefer a role second to their husbands, and this is not a position to be criticized.

There are two sides to this problem, however. There are many examples in teaching institutions of women who are carrying the responsibilities and doing the job of a particular position or office, but who are not recognized by appropriate title and rank.

"While there are some women who would just as soon 'work in the wings,' it is not true that most women *prefer* secondary roles in medicine," Dr. Lawrence states. "Most woman doctors do not want to push themselves, to demand a position or be thought of as complainers. So they do the work, and the men let them, while saying they do not want positions of responsibility."

Until more women are able to assume positions of leadership in the medical profession, there will be inhibitions against feminine progress in some areas, particularly those controlled by the conservative element in medical administration. Once her family is raised and a woman has more time to devote to her career, she can reconsider her commitment in view of the gains that could be made if she chose to assume more responsibility and helped to initiate, rather than followed, administrative policies.

Notes to Chapter Fourteen

1. Mary I. Bunting, Ph.D., "The College Years," from report of Conference on Meeting Medical Manpower Needs: The Fuller Utilization of the Woman Physician, January 12–13, 1968, Washington, D.C. Sponsored by American Medical Women's Association, President's Study Group on Careers for Women, Women's Bureau of U.S. Department of Labor. Published by American Medical Women's Association, 1968. Pp. 23–26. Reprinted by permission.
2. *Ibid.*
3. Ruth Anderson Lawrence, M.D., "The Training of Women Physicians," presented at Josiah Macy, Jr., Foundation conference on *Women for Medicine,* Dedham, Mass., October, 1966.
4. *Ibid.*
5. Carol Lopate, *Women in Medicine,* Johns Hopkins Press, 1968. P. 185.
6. *Ibid.*

Chapter Fifteen

NEW APPROACHES TO MEDICAL EDUCATION

Women who choose to study medicine as a profession are like other women in their desire for marriage and a family. However, they may need an added measure of flexibility—not of academic standards of quality but of academic timetables —if they are to combine marriage and medicine.

The battle has been won insofar as admitting women to the profession and establishing their reputation of competency. Women have made distinguished contributions to medicine for several decades and are recognized as the intellectual equals of their male peers. Intensive, flexible, individually designed programs are needed; these are not readily available in an educational system tailored for men.

If we are going to attract to medicine and make a place in the profession for the increased numbers of women clearly needed in the future, we must pay attention to some of the problems which confront a young woman who wants to become a physician. She wants to pursue a professional career which is most demanding. At the same time she has the laudable urge to build a nest and fill it with her own, and we cannot deny that this conflict often exists. We, on the other hand, need not demand that she always tackle both jobs simultaneously. The two vocations can interact, can be done in sequence if contact is maintained with the profession, or may be worked out with part-time participation.

Medical training should exploit, not eliminate, the differences between men and women. In medical school, a solution for the conflicts of the woman medical student seems to be primarily a matter of flexibility of the curriculum. We need better means of providing for prolonged leaves and for the repair of the technical obsolescence which results so rapidly. Medical education should also provide special emphasis on certain fields within medicine to which women are especially attracted, and for which they are particularly well qualified. We should give consideration to their possible needs for predictability of working schedules, and needs for mobility because of their husbands' occupations.

If we can clearly identify the unique needs and develop successful pilot programs for the training of woman physicians, we can perhaps make a contribution to medical education as important as the one which has resulted in the acceptance of women as physicians. The rigid lockstep of medical education is of concern to many medical educators. Men and women students alike need relief.

While many difficulties present themselves, they are minor indeed as compared with the faults of the alternative choices which seem to demand that most women entering medicine abandon their feminine instincts; or, to insist that only superwomen can enter medicine and no ordinary mortals need apply; or else that the physician slight both her family and professional responsibilities. None of these alternatives is a satisfactory general solution for the individual, for the public, or for the profession.[1]

Dr. Glen Leymaster, president and dean of the Woman's Medical College of Pennsylvania, thus summarized the ideal goals for educating women medical students at his inauguration in 1964. He believes that WMC, the only medical school in the country with an all-female student body, should be the pacesetter, the rallying point for all women in the profession.

Woman's Medical College

Woman's Medical College of Pennsylvania is dedicated to identifying the typically female educational problems and to innovating and experimenting with a variety of solutions. The college provides intensive, flexible, individually designed programs of a sort that are not readily available in educational systems tailored to men. WMC expects, not merely tolerates, women's problems and is experienced in solving them.

In a recent personal interview, Dr. Leymaster related WMC's progress toward the goals he set at his inauguration:

"Our efforts have been concentrated on introducing flexibility into the orthodox curriculum. Although we are not proposing radical changes in the course work, we are modifying time schedules in the classic curriculum to suit the student's individual needs. This attitude plays an important part in the success of educating the woman physician. It enables her to change schedules, examinations, and blocks of time in view of some of her other responsibilities. Pregnancy and family demands are legitimate reasons for changes here."

Dr. Leymaster is very careful to caution that educators who are sympathetic to the needs of female students should not get into the position of producing two qualities of physicians, with women the less well-trained. Every medical student should have an equal basic training. To get what she needs out of medical school, a female student must have considerable competence in math and the sciences. Some of the new medical schools give considerably less attention to everyone's doing the same thing. This trend will lead, Dr. Leymaster believes, to much less concern that all *pre*medical students study the same subjects. Even now, students are entering medical school with different majors in the sciences, rather than the traditional premedical major.

"But if the basic medical education is not the same for both women and men in medical school, we are talking about a second-rate kind of training," he warns.

"I think the question is not male-female, but whether or not each specialty, such as psychiatry, surgery, internal medicine, etc., requires the same kind of background as every other. The requirements and possible variations are being looked at, but the whole process of evaluation is in the hands of very conservative people. By consent and general application, certain prerequisites and subjects have been shown to be necessary for effective medical education. I do feel that there can be variation in the specialty training, however. Then, if a woman is more inclined to verbal skills than mathematics, she could choose psychiatry, for example."

Woman's Medical College has a policy of admitting a few older, well-qualified women after they have raised their families, although this policy is considered to carry a far greater risk than the conventional one of limiting acceptance to girls in their early twenties. The college currently is not admitting as many older students as in its earlier days because the number of highly qualified younger women in the applicant pool has greatly increased.

"In general, we recognize this policy as risky, in terms of the older woman's not completing medical school or dropping out of the profession later. We have admitted a few nurses and some older women with children because we felt they had particular attributes that would compensate for the risk. They have been quite successful, but the attrition rate is higher," Dr. Leymaster says.

Woman's Medical College keeps an open mind, however, and the talented older woman will get a hearing, whereas she usually would not be considered by the majority of medical schools in the United States. As elsewhere, the present limitations at WMC are of faculty and space, not of prospective students. As these problems are eased, it is expected that the attraction of other careers may cause shortages of qualified students in many medical schools. At that time, Dr. Leymaster believes, the growing interest of women in careers in medicine will be of critical national importance.

WMC has embarked on an ambitious program to rehabilitate its physical facilities, is trying to make maximum use of its faculty resources, and has strengthened its departments of pediatrics, psychiatry, and physiology—specialties that strongly attract woman physicians. The college is having financial problems in implementing its plans, since it is not part of a state educational system or university and must rely on private endowments. Scholarship funds for undergraduate students of limited means are urgently needed, as are stipends for intensive postgraduate study for women returning to professional work after a period devoted to raising a family. Details of the WMC Continuing Education Program appear in Chapter 18.

Tutorial Programs

Several medical schools have instituted tutorial programs, using their existing faculties to provide counseling and individualized curriculum planning for students. This workable and sensible approach permits a wide latitude of experience for each individual within the school's established framework of courses. Each first- and second-year student is assigned a faculty tutor who establishes a personal relationship with him on a one-to-one ratio. This service is beneficial for both men and women, and it is not suggested that such an approach be limited to women.

Depending on individual preferences, a student can be given an opportunity to do research in his field of interest, or acquire an early familiarization with clinical medicine. The tutor guides the student's training and career choices and tries to make sure that his goals are realistic. This is a good way of warning the woman who may be biting off more than she can chew in terms of professional responsibilities that later could conflict with her family duties. Most of the female students are assigned to woman faculty members, when possible to those who are mothers. One director of such a program believes that every medical school should expose its young woman students to faculty member-mothers at some time during their early years.

Girls must be aware that they should seek counsel beyond the college level. With the new flexibility being introduced into medical school curricula across the country, suitable schedules can be worked out to meet varying needs, provided the girl is aware of all the possibilities. More and more schools are permitting an increasing number of electives, because of the tremendous amount of material that has to be presented. Previously, in the rigidly structured courses of medical study, a female student attracted unfavorable attention if she did not take particular subjects at a particular time or complete everything when her classmates did. Both male and female students benefit from being able to arrange their schedules to suit individual needs, and now a girl "can elect to have a baby" during one semester without losing out in her overall training, as one faculty member put it.

Northwestern University's Honors Program

In 1961, Northwestern University Medical School initiated a revolutionary curriculum designed to meet the growing competition with other professions for talented students. One of the aims of the program is to "provide gifted students with additional incentive to enter the field of medicine"—an open recognition of the fact that the space-age physical sciences are attracting many of the nation's top scholars away from medicine, despite some official protestations to the contrary.

In place of the traditional sharp division between premedical and medical education, Northwestern's Honors Program offers an integrated curriculum combining course material from the college of arts and sciences, the medical school, and the graduate school over the six-year study span. The college-level material has been redesigned to include science courses that have a more direct bearing on the study of medicine. The humanities, in the form of seminar discussions, are carried into the final years of the program.

The university was aware that a single solution for all students preparing for medicine "was neither desirable nor possible" and decided to concentrate its efforts on a program for the most promising students who had prepared in the most advanced high schools. It was believed that the program "could later be broadened as experience was gained. A challenging and exciting opportunity might reduce the loss of the most capable students to other disciplines." [2]

For this reason, the program is not suitable as a model for most medical students; the participants are in the upper 3 percent of their high school graduating classes, with almost half of those accepted at the very top of their classes.[3] However, several features of the program are applicable to all schools that wish to provide more realistic premedical education. Of particular relevance is the integration of course work at all levels.

Northwestern found that the introduction of special science courses into its medical Honors Program stimulated the biology department into revising completely its curriculum for biology majors. The concept of an integrated sequence of science training, with each new course heavily relying on material from the previous courses, is now a regular offering of the college of arts and sciences with the result that the Honors Program students no longer require special science courses but take the departmental sequence.

This better preparation has made it possible for the first year of the medical school curriculum to be completely revised and the second year significantly modified. Thus, a fresh approach originated for a small group of students has had far-reaching influence throughout the university.

Another feature of the program's flexibility is the opportunity to earn a Ph.D. degree as well as an M.D. The combined degrees permit students to prepare for careers in academic medicine or medical research along with the practice of medicine. Students who elect this course of study must take an additional two or three years; they can enter the program at the end of their second year. Those who take the six-year program qualify for a Bachelor of Science degree at the end of four years and are awarded the M.D. at the end of six years. A student may leave the program at any time without penalty; some change their minds concerning their ultimate careers and switch to fields other than medicine. Two or three per year, out of the approximately thirty selected, run into serious scholastic problems and are transferred to other academic areas in the university. A student may spend an additional year in the college of arts and sciences without losing his place in the medical school, or may decide to take the traditional eight-year path if the accelerated course proves to be too much of a burden.

Research training is available as a voluntary activity which, at the student's option, may be added to the regular curriculum. The aim of the Research Training Program is to provide students with a practical background in research and enable them to make career decisions based on firsthand knowledge rather than on advice and intuition. Each student participating in the program is awarded a twelve-week research fellowship to be used during the summer months, beginning with the summer following completion of the first year. The fellowship provides a stipend of six hundred dollars and gives the student an opportunity to conduct laboratory research under the preceptorship of an experienced and active investigator.

Faculty members who have worked with the Honors Program students have reported that it was enormously satisfying and challenging. Some who criticized the program in its early stages predicted that the science faculty would be unwilling to participate in the special courses. Not only have these predictions been proved incorrect, but the course revisions have resulted in new approaches to teaching throughout the university. The new science courses are considered a particularly desirable teaching assignment, and in fact they have been used as an inducement in recruiting new faculty members.

The success of the accelerated curriculum is described by Allen Lein, Ph.D., director of the Honors Program:

"Although the Honors Program began as an experiment, it is now an ongoing and significant part of the University's educational operation, and is considered by most of the participating faculty to be an unqualified success." [4]

The performance of the students has been most gratifying. "Although it is not employed for selection purposes, students in the Honors Program are asked to take the MCAT at the end of their second year, just prior to registration in the Medical School. In each category, and without exception, the Honors students have achieved scores higher than those of their classmates, in spite of the fact that they have had only two years of college. . . . The scores of the Honors students average over 50 points higher than those of the others." [5]

To date, thirty-five girls have been enrolled in the program. Of that number, twenty are currently registered in some phase of the program, four have received their M.D.'s and are taking their internships or residencies, and eleven are no longer enrolled in the program.[6]

If you are interested in such a program, you should work toward it from the outset of your high school education. Participants are selected during their senior year in high school; therefore, early application and preparation are essential. One of the most satisfying features of such a program is that it enables a student to progress through premed studies with the assurance of a seat in medical school.

Northwestern considers itself well rewarded for its efforts at innovation. The success of the Honors Program "has served to create an atmosphere of inquiry and ferment and to loosen the hold of traditional and time-worn educational methods. It has brought about reexamination of the undergraduate programs in science in the College of Arts and Sciences and has furnished an important link between the two campuses of the University. Through discussions, the faculty has a better understanding of the needs and challenges offered by educating bright students in the life sciences." [7]

Boston University's Six-Year Program

Boston University has developed a six-year program similar to that of Northwestern. It offers a combined curriculum designed to improve the quality of medical education while shortening the overall period of study. Students are admitted to the college of liberal arts and the school of medicine simultaneously upon graduation from high school.

The first two years are devoted to premedical studies in the college of liberal arts. Classes are small, the majority are at honors level, and most of the courses have been developed specifically for the program. Three summer sessions are included, with adequate time for vacation, to complete the liberal arts requirements. At the end of the second year, each student has a reevaluation interview to determine whether he has the maturity and emotional stability necessary for promotion into the third year of the program. First-year medical studies begin in this third year, and the amount of time devoted to medical courses remains the same as in the conventional program. Liberal arts and medical courses are interrelated to eliminate repetitive material. Upon successful conpletion of the program, students are awarded the degrees of Bachelor of Arts and Doctor of Medicine.

In Boston's program emphasis is placed on small-group instruction; there are small classes, seminars, and tutorials. Electives are available each year, and the final summer is devoted entirely to electives, from which the student is required to select a minor. A student who, for any reason (academic, motivational, or emotional), is found to be ill-suited for the program may be transferred without loss of credits into the regular liberal arts curriculum. Upon graduation, such students may continue with their medical education by the conventional route. Students also may voluntarily transfer from the program at any point and continue their liberal arts education at Boston University or elsewhere.

Boston's six-year program is now entering its eighth year. Half of the last two classes of medical students to be graduated have been composed of students in the program.

Dean Franklin G. Ebaugh, Jr., reports on the program's success to date:

> Based on the evaluation of the last two graduating classes, the six-year students performed in every way comparable to the students who took eight years to complete their undergraduate and medical education insofar as performance on National Boards, internal grading, quality of Internships obtained, participation in extracurricular school activities such as election to student honors, equal number of officers elected to Student Council and to offices of various student organizations, equal participation in student activities, such as the Year Book, Newspaper, etc.
>
> In short, we can find no difference in the performance or the characteristics of the six-year students by the time they have graduated from Medical School.[8]

This program, like Northwestern's, is designed for the superior achiever. The school states that "applicants must present evidence of academic achievement of high quality and should have received College Entrance Examination Board Scholastic Aptitude Test scores in the top 10 percent of national distribution." [9]

The curriculum is greatly accelerated and well-suited for the gifted young woman who is determined to complete her medical education before she marries and begins her family. The summer schedules are particularly heavy as compared to the average load carried in summer school; fifteen credits must be completed in two six-week sessions. The student must take nine credits during at least one summer session, and only a superior intellect can manage such a load.

As now designed, these accelerated combination programs are not the solution for the majority of students who are seeking greater flexibility. Also, they represent no drastic change in the medical school curriculum, but rather are a telescoping of the traditional training. Accelerated programs have the advantage of eliminating most of the overlapping in course material that exists in the conventional eight-year system, since the six-year curriculum is designed specifically for the program as a whole, with each subsequent course building on the one preceding it.

Curriculum variations are being initiated at many of the new medical schools, and students should study them carefully before deciding to apply. The trend toward more variety and flexibility is just beginning in medical schools. The student must be able to distinguish programs that suit his personal goals from those that do not. Many medical schools offer the opportunity to study for the Ph.D. and the M.D. simultaneously; such a program is advantageous to the student preparing for a career in research or teaching.

Curriculum Revision and Innovation

A number of established medical schools are breaking with tradition and initiating totally new concepts of medical education. This is a positive but often a difficult undertaking, as existing course material must be evaluated carefully and many administrators and faculty members won over.

Modern scientific advances make it mandatory to reexamine medical training. The explosion of medical and scientific knowledge during the past few decades has made it virtually impossible to continue attempting to teach every medical student the entire body of medical knowledge. Moreover, the traditional curricula of most medical schools in the United States have not changed significantly from the turn of the century. Another source of dissatisfaction is that the rigid structure of the conventional curriculum does not recognize the differing interests, background preparation, and career goals of individual students.

The Curriculum Committee of the University of Miami (Florida) School of Medicine has recently completed a two-year study of what the members considered was an outdated curriculum. Their findings resulted in the introduction in 1968 of a program of contemporary medical training with innovations at every level. In addition to the work of the committee and of several faculty subcommittees, the students were invited to contribute toward the revision by pointing out the weaknesses and strengths of the teaching program. The students also led the fight for a complete reevaluation of the school's grading system.

These combined efforts resulted in the following statement of objectives:

"The new curriculum must be very flexible to provide for the variety of requirements and challenges present in modern medicine. The previous concept that each student must be required to take the same courses has been abandoned herewith." [10]

Considerable time is being provided for electives, with the total to vary according to the ultimate career interests of the individual. There will be fewer straight lectures, less factual information will be presented, and much less memorization will be required of the students. "An effort must be made to encourage a graduate school environment in the true sense and to discourage the present trade school philosophies." Free time will be scheduled each week, to allow the students to read, reflect, and digest what they are learning. Emphasis will be placed on the learning of concepts rather than the memorization of details.

The first two years of Miami's new medical program contain a basic core curriculum to which all students will be exposed. "Emphasis in these courses is placed as much as possible on the use of conceptual tools and not on the dissemination of details." [11] Instead of the conventional blocks of subjects scheduled at a specific time of the year and the teaching of the basic sciences as individual disciplines, they are being treated as integrated subject matter in interdisciplinary courses and in correlation with clinical processes.

Freshman students will be introduced at the outset of their schooling to clinical medicine, the patient, and the ward setting. Clinical correlation conferences are scheduled each week to relate the preclinical training to the student's goal of becoming a practicing physician. A 22 percent reduction in the time allocated to the basic sciences permits this early introduction to clinical teaching. The number of small-group teaching conferences has been increased during the first two years, and time is allowed for study prior to the examination periods.

Similar revisions are being carried into the second year. Interdepartmental subjects are taught, and didactic lectures and laboratory time have been drastically reduced (by more than 20 percent). A new clinical cancer training program has been introduced into the second semester.

Sophomore students are divided into small groups and are taught to do patient histories and physical examinations under the careful supervision of a single faculty member. Students also are taught how to perform psychiatric interviews. Problem solving and the physician-patient relationship are emphasized.

The clinical years have undergone some revolutionary changes. There are no regular summer vacations. Clinical clerks begin two straight years of teaching in August, although a student may elect to take a month's vacation each year. When clerkships in the required core clinical curriculum are completed, the student enters a structured elective program that provides opportunities for a variety of careers in medicine. The broadly based program can be divided into clinical and research electives. Students may elect to spend some time at other medical institutions. This phase of the program is still under study, and various new electives are being developed, many of which will reintroduce the basic sciences in combination with the clinical electives. Advanced courses and seminars will also be offered.

The Adviser System. The new modified curriculum with its emphasis on a flexible elective program is reinforced by a new active advisory system. Each faculty member is assigned four medical students, whom he counsels throughout their medical education. Emphasis is placed on personal and academic problems, choice of electives, and formation of career goals. The faculty member will not be assigned any additional students until his original freshmen have graduated.

Proposed Three-Year Medical Curriculum. The university's medical school Curriculum Committee hopes that the modified curriculum presently being taught will lead to an even more imaginative revision. Now under consideration is a plan that would both shorten the formal medical school program and provide the student with a fourth-year university internship.

The proposed program does not necessitate a drastic reduction of preclinical time; rather, it recommends a more efficient use of the time previously allocated to excessive and unimaginative laboratory exercises. Instead of a twenty-week vacation each academic year, the student would be permitted eight weeks of free time annually. When one considers that by this time most of a medical student's peers will have graduated from college and will have jobs that permit only two-week annual vacations, the reasoning behind this reduction becomes apparent. When the tedious memorization of detail is reduced, the long vacation relief traditionally required by the beleaguered student is no longer necessary.

"Forty weeks of clinical training would follow the preclinical course. This would be more flexible than past programs in that the students would not be required to take all of the clinical specialties. Finally, students would be offered 30 weeks of clinical electives integrated with basic sciences."

After completion of the proposed three-year program (which contains virtually the same number of course hours as the present revised curriculum) several alternatives would be available:

"Some students would be required to take a fourth year. Most could receive their M.D. degrees after a year of approved internship. Hopefully, the majority of students would enter a University of Miami-supervised internship and residency program which would be a natural extension of the three-year curriculum.

"This program, coupled with admission of qualified three-year premedical students, could reduce by two years the present eight years needed to obtain the M.D. degree. More importantly, it would provide the student with a more realistic basis from which to continue medical training." [12]

Notes to Chapter Fifteen

1. Glen R. Leymaster, M.D., "Tomorrow's Target," inaugural address as President and Dean of Woman's Medical College of Pennsylvania, March 6, 1964.
2. John A. D. Cooper, M.D., and Allen Lein, Ph.D., "An Integrated Program for Premedical and Medical Education: Its Impact on the University," *Journal of Mount Sinai Hospital*, Vol. 34, No. 3, May-June 1967.
3. *Ibid.*
4. Personal communication from Mrs. B. L. Borr, secretary to Allen Lein,

Ph.D., Director of Honors Program in Medical Education, Northwestern University, Chicago, Ill., July 23, 1968.
5. Cooper and Lein, *op. cit.*
6. Borr, *op. cit.*
7. Cooper and Lein, *op. cit.*
8. Personal communication from Dean Franklin G. Ebaugh, Jr., Boston University, July 15, 1968.
9. *Six-Year Program in Liberal Arts and Medicine,"* Boston University, Boston, Mass., 1968.
10. *The Status of Curriculum Revision at the University of Miami School of Medicine,* University of Miami, Florida, September, 1968.
11. *Ibid.*
12. *Ibid.*

Chapter Sixteen

EXPANSION OF MEDICAL EDUCATIONAL FACILITIES

Expansion of existing educational facilities is the most urgent need facing the medical profession in the United States today. The physician shortage cannot be alleviated until there is a means of educating additional doctors. The lack of seats in medical schools forecloses the opportunity of studying medicine to many qualified students, men and women alike. The most convincing argument of those who would like to limit the number of woman physicians is: "Women are taking up enough of the men's seats already." Those who believe that expansion should come before recruiting tend to agree.

The opportunity to study medicine should be available to every student who demonstrates the combination of qualities that point toward successful completion of training and service to humanity. For decades, medical education in this country has been limited because of a refusal to increase enrollment in existing medical schools, and because of delays in establishing new schools by the private sector of the medical community.

In a face of an overwhelming physician shortage and public awareness of the reasons for it, government funds and a limited amount of private investment have been channeled into expansion efforts. Only with continued government support can this expansion be maintained. An informed public must be aware of how crucial this support is to its own health and well-being.

Dr. David Denker, President of New York Medical College, has launched an effort to expand the enrollment of the school by 100 percent and has issued a call to other established medical schools to do the same. He and other leaders in medical education see a great discrepancy between the type of advanced medical care that research is making possible and the actual care that is available to most of the world's population.

"The crisis of today is not one of knowledge. It is a crisis of responsibility and of social philosophy, a crisis stigmatized by inadequacy and unavailability. What we have is in short supply, and too few of us can get at it. We are crowding ourselves away from our own banquet table. A world confronted by an exploding population is further confounded by a second crisis of scientists in shortage. Central to this scientist shortage is the massive doctor deficit." [1]

The effort to supply more educational facilities to meet our ever-expanding population must be a continuing process. We cannot open a few medical schools which produce an additional one hundred or two hundred physicians per year, and then sit back smugly thinking the crisis has been met. Nor can we leave it to the next generation to alleviate the shortage.

"These are *our* times, and the problems of today are *our* own problems," Dr. Denker asserts. "The class which graduates this year will be practicing medicine in the year 2000. The men and women trained today will also be teaching and researching in the year 2000. So, the facilities we build tomorrow must be relevant to the year 2000 and to an estimated population of 6 billion 400 million." [2]

The number of medical school applicants will continue to exceed the number of those accepted in the next few decades; yet every qualified applicant is urgently needed. This state of affairs suggests, Dr. Denker points out, that our doctor deficit does not result from a lack of available or qualified young men and women interested in medicine, but rather both from a deficiency in those who are responsible for student admissions at each medical school and from the inadequate number of medical schools in the country. Each person entering the profession should keep informed about the medical crisis in the United States and resolve to support efforts to educate greater numbers of physicians.

"We must find new ways to expand and teach more medical students. The pressure on the profession will become so great that the schools will have to respond. Our aspiration here at New York

Medical College is to double our number of graduates as quickly as we can while still maintaining quality."

"Pressure on the profession" is a significant phrase. It points up the responsibility of every individual concerned with improving medical care to make his opinions heard.

The American Medical Association now favors an increased number of seats in medical school classes. Dr. Hayden C. Nicholson, director of the Department of Undergraduate Medical Education of the AMA, says:

"The American Medical Association is very much concerned about the shortage of physicians in the United States. However, the shortage can be attributed more to lack of facilities in American medical schools than to lack of qualified students interested in the study of medicine. Considerable progress is being made in expanding medical educational facilities. About fifteen medical schools have recently been established or are in process of being established.

"In the past, about half the medical schools in the country have been private schools and the other half governmental schools, usually state schools. However, almost all the schools being established now are governmentally supported. There is no question that the availability of federal funds, both for construction and for operations, has been an important factor in the establishment of new schools and the expansion of existing ones. Medical education has become very expensive. Private funds are still very important in the support of medical education, but there is no doubt that such education is becoming increasingly dependent upon governmental funds, local, state, and federal." [3]

Most medical educators agree that it takes too long to build new schools. Dr. Denker provides the example of one eastern medical school that took fourteen years to develop and recently opened with sixteen students; they will ultimately have only sixty-seven. Dr. Nicholson concurs: "It is true that a long time elapses between the decision to establish a new medical school and the time when the graduates of that school are exerting a significant impact upon the availability of medical care." [4]

Insufficient medical schools and inadequate teaching facilities are the bottleneck in American medical education today. But Mary Dublin Keyserling, former director of the Women's Bureau of the United States Department of Labor, believes that the expansion of medical training facilities is on the way.

"The output of existing medical schools, we are told, at presently planned levels, will provide about 360,000 physicians by 1975 as compared with the 400,000 goal set forth in recent manpower reports. It is not unlikely that we will lift this training schedule because we, in the United States, do have a way of meeting urgent unmet needs once they are made clear. And our needs for medical manpower are very clear." [5]

Mrs. Keyserling believes that "there will be sufficient increase to warrant changes in our approach to the counseling and guidance of our young women and girls, starting at the very early years when self-image is established. If more women are . . . to realize their potentials . . . they need to have wider areas of choice. And the time to begin is now."

It is expected that the opening of new medical schools and the increased enrollments planned by many existing schools will raise the number of new physicians from the eight thousand graduated in 1967 to a number significantly near the target of twelve thousand annually within the next few years. [6]

The interacting problems of lack of physical facilities and shortage of medical teaching personnel illustrate how medicine has bred its own conundrum: How do you train more doctors to teach more doctors when you don't have the facilities to train more doctors?

"It seems clear that a medical school requires three things besides students: namely, an adequate faculty, the laboratories and supporting facilities to teach the basic preclinical sciences, and a system of giving health care, usually a hospital, in which students can learn and observe the actual practice of medicine. It is difficult to come by all of these facilities at the present time. We need both to expand existing facilities to their limits and to build new schools. We need a more conscientious and intelligent involvement by society—taxes will probably be the solution." Dr. James Bartlett, associate dean of the University of Rochester School of Medicine, delineates the problem, and adds that women have a major contribution to make in relieving the medical faculty shortage.

"The construction of new health educational facilities is in the nature of the building of a national resource and beyond the capacity of private gifts and voluntary contributions. Even with sufficient money, sufficient bricks and mortar, and the scientific and health care facilities required for a medical school, we will still have a problem in the shortage of faculty members. There are great needs for people in every aspect of medicine today and the growth of new schools requires more and more teachers in medicine." [7]

In addition to recruiting more physicians and Ph.D.'s in the medical sciences into academic medicine, we can make use of the highly trained personnel already available who are not teaching, as well as finding better ways of utilizing our current faculty members.

Dr. Denker has some specific solutions: "The emphasis must be on innovative techniques that will take the burden off the faculty. A two-track system can be utilized; that is, we can set up two separate faculties—one drawn from the very valuable group consisting of recently retired doctors. These people can make a real contribution. Retired doctors might serve as tutors in the clinical years of medical education when a small student-teacher ratio is required. Then additional full-time faculty members could be used for the preclinical years to permit an increase in students. We must also revise the curriculum in ways that would take advantage of such a flexible, two-track system."

The financial compensations as well as the intellectual satisfactions of research attract many of the finest scientific minds away from teaching, at least a large proportion of the time. When deciding how to apportion his available working hours, a young doctor should consider the most urgent needs of the profession in addition to his personal requirements. To break the cycle of insufficient faculty resulting in too few medical school graduates each year, more teachers are needed immediately. Those who divide their time between teaching and research could evaluate their contribution earnestly; many faculty members admit privately that they have additional hours available for instruction.

"The faculty could be used a lot more efficiently right now," one professor stated vehemently. "I could do ten times more teaching if I devoted my whole time to it, considerably more even if I didn't teach full-time. Some courses take only four months out of the year."

"The worst part of the whole thing," he continued, "is that research and patients are more exciting intellectually. More rewarding. They distract you from the students, particularly after a number of years."

The ideal solution, both administrators and concerned teachers say, would be not to permit full-time faculty members to do research or take private patients. Such restrictions, however, would make it difficult to attract top-quality teachers. The better qualified faculty, particularly the male members, derive a great deal of satisfaction and prestige from research and would not accept teaching appointments if their investigations were curtailed. In the clinical years, most of the actual teaching is done by volunteers who come in a few hours a week to teach their specialties, one educator pointed out. It is the preclinical instructors in the basic medical sciences who must be utilized to the utmost, and here women can play a decisive role.

"I don't agree that people [faculty members] are not busy enough," says Dr. Glen Leymaster, president of Woman's Medical College of Pennsylvania. "But teaching does not have as high a priority as research in terms of the need. There is a question of priority; some could teach more if they did not do as much research; this is the competitive thing in terms of time. This means that less research would be one way of increasing the needed teaching time.

"The other activities that compete with time for teaching are things that should be done, that is, the time spent teaching allied . . . health personnel, and the time spent taking care of patients. There aren't enough doctors to take care of the patients now."

Dr. George Lewis, associate dean of the University of Miami (Florida) School of Medicine, hopes that a de-emphasis of government support for medical research may channel some of the highly trained scientific specialists now working on grants into faculty positions in the medical schools:

"In order to expand medical facilities and train more medical students, we first must have more teachers. In the last ten years, the biggest problem has been the decided emphasis on training of research people, on an increasing number of Ph.D.'s, and not teachers.

"Financial assistance, particularly from the federal government, has been for research. Why should a doctor go into the teaching profession when this is not where fame and fortune lie? If he wants to go up in his profession, he does not go into teaching. The government must give more assistance to medical educators. Lately, the amount of money in project research has begun to "dry up" and this may start a new trend. We have turned out Ph.D.'s by the score, who are trained to research, and these people look toward the federal government to support them in their programs. If the government has no money to set them up in a research career, hopefully they will turn to teaching."

Dr. Denker also hopes that a new trend is being established— one which will instill a greater idea of service, both to the patient and the profession. "We have been producing doctors who are extraordinary technicians, but many of them are limited in their understanding of our culture. But society is now demanding greater relevance between education of physicians and the needs of our citizens. The ideal physician, like the ideal teacher, should be trained in the "human skills." He should feel a responsibility to help improve the conditions under which men live. The generation of doctors now being trained appears to have more social awareness and a greater sense of involvement than has generally been seen in the medical profession."

Linked to the necessity of providing sufficient facilities to train all of the talented Americans who desire to study medicine is the need to produce enough physicians to supply our nation and therefore stop the drain on foreign talent. Our refusal to provide enough seats in medical school to educate the physicians we require has created such a shortage of doctors that thousands of internships and residencies in this country are being filled each year by graduates of medical schools abroad—often from countries that can least afford to lose them. Instead of providing help for countries that desperately need to improve health services for their own people, we are draining their already pitifully short supply of medical personnel.

In Dr. Denker's words:

"The poorest nations, those in greatest need, are losing their already woefully inadequate number of scientists, specialists, doctors, and technicians to wealthier lands, including our own . . . surely we should be maximizing our training and reordering our training structure, not merely to meet the needs of American science and society, but to assuage, rather than aggravate, the scientific manpower shortage of less fortunate societies.

"Whereas we should be proudly exporting our medical skills and talents to Latin America, Africa, and Asia, we are instead siphoning their sorely needed doctors into our medical economy. In effect, poorly developed countries are today subsidizing our medical manpower pool.

". . . the training we give foreign doctors and medical students is more applicable to our own medical problems, and our own system of medical care, than it is related to the problems and needs of their native lands. So, often it all ends up with the foreign physicians never returning to their native lands, but staying on in our comparatively affluent medical economy. This is not good. It is not healthy. It is not right."

Dr. Denker points out how medical schools in the United States could help reverse this trend:

"All medical institutions have the obligation to increase the total number of doctors at least 100% and make available much higher proportions of medical personnel to countries which sorely lack doctors.

"We should reorient the medical curriculum to turn out graduates who will be equipped and trained to work in the countries where they must work. . . . A medical student from an underdeveloped country who is trained in the United States in diagnostic techniques will not be prepared for the conditions he finds when he is sent back home. . . . [We should] establish programs abroad to reorient medical students, particularly in the less developed countries. [We should] also help them work closely with their colleagues at home to produce more medical students." [8]

The physician shortage in the United States has far-reaching effects. Taking the international view, our affluent nation must not only provide the doctors we need for our own citizens, but help, rather than hinder, health care development throughout the world.

Notes to Chapter Sixteen

1. David Denker, Ph.D., "Cultural Crisis of Our Time: The Medical Revolution and the Alarming Doctor Shortage," installation address as President of New York Medical College, published in *Chironian Magazine*, New York Medical College, Winter, 1967–68.
2. *Ibid.*
3. Personal communication from Hayden C. Nicholson, M.D., Director of Division of Medical Education, American Medical Association, September 19, 1968. Statistics published in *Journal of the American Medical Association*, November, 1968.
4. *Ibid.*
5. Mary Dublin Keyserling, "Concluding Remarks: Conference Summary," from report of a conference on Meeting Medical Manpower Needs: The Fuller Utilization of the Woman Physician, January 12–13, 1968, Washington, D.C. Sponsored by American Medical Women's Association, President's Study Group on Careers for Women, Women's Bureau of U.S. Department of Labor. Published by American Medical Women's Association, 1968. P. 80. Reprinted by permission.
6. *Ibid.*

7. Personal communication from James W. Bartlett, M.D., Associate Dean, University of Rochester School of Medicine, Rochester, N.Y., January 19, 1967.
8. Denker, *op. cit.*

Chapter Seventeen

POSTGRADUATE PROGRAMS WITH NEW FLEXIBILITY

"In recruiting talent for medicine, the feminine half of American brainpower is being ignored. It is quite possible that the need for more physicians can only be met if a larger number of women are attracted to medicine as a career. But beyond the quantitative problem is the fact that women enter fields of medicine, such as pediatrics and child and adolescent psychiatry, that are urgently in need of physicians. The medical schools and the teaching hospitals should face up to the question, 'Should there be a higher percentage of women entering medicine?' If the answer is 'yes'—and I suggest that it should be—these institutions must take positive steps to attract larger numbers of women and make it possible for them (despite the added responsibilities of marriage and motherhood) to complete their training, including the internship and residency." [1]

Macy Foundation Program: Women for Medicine

The author of the above quotation, Dr. John Z. Bowers, is president of the Josiah Macy, Jr., Foundation, a philanthropic organization with headquarters in New York City, whose policy is "to initiate, stimulate, develop, and support scientific investigations of the fundamental aspects of health, of sickness, and of methods for the relief of suffering." [2] The foundation's funds are pledged "for the architecture of men and ideas" rather than for the building of facilities. The programs the foundation administers are pioneer efforts in improvement and innovation rather than implementation of the status quo.

Because the United States has one of the lowest percentages of women in medicine in the world today, the Macy Foundation convened a conference on the subject at Dedham, Massachusetts, in October of 1966. Some of the major topics discussed at the conference have been examined in previous chapters. The conclusions that resulted from this national gathering of medical educational brainpower are: (a) We need women in medicine—"about 50 percent of our potential brainpower is neglected—untapped for medicine"; and (b) "There are fields in which the woman physician can make a unique contribution." [3]

"One approach to the problem of attracting more talented women for medicine is to demonstrate the possibility for a woman to continue training after medical school while at the same time filling her role as wife and mother." [4] As important as the need for attracting more women to medicine is the need to utilize our women in medicine after they have completed their training. The Macy Foundation is supporting programs that will allow women who have graduated from medical school to make maximum contributions to medicine.

The Radcliffe Program. In July, 1966, the Macy Foundation made a four-year grant in the amount of $100,000 to the Radcliffe Institute for Independent Study. The purpose of the grant was to assist woman physicians in the Boston area to continue their graduate training, and in some cases to reenter medical practice through refresher training.

In the 1966–1967 program there were fourteen individual grants ranging from one thousand dollars to three thousand dollars, four for students in medical school and ten for postgraduate training. In the 1967–1968 program, Macy funds went to fourteen residents and seven other fellows. The recipients may use the funds for any expenses incurred in continuing their education, including child care and household help. Traditionally, grants have been awarded only to full-time students or residents, usually earmarked for tuition and sometimes living allowances.

The Radcliffe groups should make excellent subjects for the evaluation of so broad and versatile an approach to the problems of the woman physician. Will funds alone answer the problem of keeping women in medicine? "Over half of our woman physicians are married to men in the most affluent profession in the United States—medicine." [5] Flexible scheduling rather than cash awards may be the success factor in the Macy approach, as the Foundation is supporting only programs that offer extended or part-time training. The recipients of the grants are well-qualified young women, all of whom "are strongly motivated, and ready to make substantial sacrifices for their careers." [6]

President Mary I. Bunting of Radcliffe has reported that "in a number of cases the Macy funds are literally the key to the continuation of medical training; in other cases the money enables a young physician to provide properly, rather than haphazardly, for the care of her children while she is at the school or at the hospital." [7]

Simple statistics on the number of female physicians married to male physicians do not give the complete financial picture, however. A young female physician married to an intern or resident would not be in a position of sufficient affluence to continue her career at the expense of her husband's training. It would be the mother-physician, not the male, who would drop out of medicine. Therefore, funding at this critical stage in the life of a newly established family may be the only means of keeping the woman in the profession.

Other Macy Foundation Grants. A grant has been made by the Macy Foundation to Stanford University Medical Center, primarily for graduate programs for woman physicians, on the basis of the willingness of the departments of psychiatry, anesthesiology, and internal medicine to develop less-than-full-time residency programs for women. A grant has also been made to Woman's Medical College of Pennsylvania for a graduate and postgraduate training program for woman physicians. This program is described in the next chapter.

New York Medical College Psychiatric
Residency Training Program

In 1962, the department of psychiatry of the New York Medical College introduced an innovation in the graduate training of woman physicians with children. It is called the psychiatric training program for physician-mothers. The college recognized that the conflict between domestic and professional duties caused most of the difficulties for young married women in postgraduate training programs in medicine. In setting out to do something to alleviate the situation, NYMC became a pacesetter for the nation. The first step in inititating any totally new concept in education is to recognize and define the problem. "The current long and rigidly structured postgraduate medical training programs were developed for men by men with little recognition of the needs of women and, specifically, of women with small children. A woman's conflicts are aggravated because the period of residency training usually coincides chronologically with a woman's child-raising years." [8]

Inspiration for the pioneer program came from Dr. Helen Kaplan, who had married before she entered medical school. Dr. Kaplan had her first baby six days before her medical school classes started, her second during her senior year, and her third during her residency.

"Medical school was not bad," Dr. Kaplan reminisces. "I first ran into conflicts between duties and home demands during my internship, when I was required to live in the hospital." She realized that there was no good reason for the inflexibility of internship, that the night and weekend duty was not essential for training, although it was for service. Dr. Kaplan began to think about ways in which flexibility could be introduced into such training and applied them to her residency. Her husband, Dr. Harold Kaplan, is chief of the psychiatric education and training program at New York Medical College, and he, together with Dr. Alfred Freedman, chairman of the department, and Dr. Clifford Sager, chief of clinical services of the department, created what is now known as the "mother's program."

"My husband's initial reaction was very favorable when I told him of our ideas. I was fortunate that we began our program in a department headed by men who like women to make a contribution. The people in authority were in favor of our suggestion from the outset.

"Instead of just a modification in the time of my own training, I wanted to make this an institutional policy. I felt the opportunity should be available to any qualified mother with the same needs—who does not want to give up either motherhood or her profession."

Dr. Kaplan believes that competitiveness between men and women originally led to the traditional attitude that rigid training is a "part of the price you have to pay to get into the union." As conditions now exist, a woman "has to pay a terrible price." Dr. Kaplan points out that there is an emotional investment in any institution, and medical training has a long tradition.

"There is a great emotional investment in this tradition of inflexibility, of dedication to service. It boils down to a realization that men do not like women in the field; it *is* a competitive field. They went through it, and feel others should, too. If you remove all these obstacles, then you no longer make it so special, so difficult. They are afraid then that 'anyone could do it.' "

It is Dr. Kaplan's opinion that when you define your goals rationally, you can see the real needs without the emotion.

There are good reasons for being constantly available to patients, and these valid reasons brought about the tradition in medicine of selfless dedication and personal sacrifice. At one time, residents could not marry. Such considerations, however, are not essential to good training, Dr. Kaplan believes.

"Define the purpose of the residency," she says. "The residency is to train people who can make a greater contribution. It does not *require* rigid training."

The Kaplans believed that a flexible program could play a particularly important role in the specialty of psychiatry. Psychiatry and child psychiatry are among the top choices of women who specialize, yet the vast potential supply of practitioners has barely been tapped in this country because so few women enter medicine. The loss of women to medicine, the Kaplans reasoned, naturally affects psychiatry, a field that has an acute shortage of physicians and can ill afford to lose any female recruits to its increasingly insufficient ranks.

The department of psychiatry agreed and has supported the program in the belief that women have made and have yet to make many valuable and unique contributions to the specialty. To encourage their entry into this field, the program was launched.

Extended training. An important feature of this residency for mother-physicians is that it offers "modified-time" training, not part-time. The desirability of this type of schedule and the failure of several part-time attempts will be evaluated in the next chapter.

"Resident mothers work 'full-time'—that is, from 9 A.M. to 5 P.M.—and also serve emergency night duty. Although they work nine months during each year, the three months they do not work are made up at the end of their training by an additional nine months' training period. Thus, the mothers require four calendar years to complete their training." [9]

This modification in the time sequences gives the mother a more normal family life and enables her to spend important time with her young children. The resident-mother commits herself to four nine-month periods, usually beginning on September 1 instead of July 1, as most hospital training programs require.

The mother spends summer vacations with her children and is given time off at Christmas and at Easter. Although some mothers elect to work longer periods, perhaps ten or eleven months per year, none may work for less than nine months per year.

Mother-residents are assigned enough night duty to meet the demands of good training and the standards of the American Board of Psychiatry, but there are modifications in their schedules and also in their weekend duty assignments. They participate fully in all the classroom and clinical activities of the department's regular residency program. Therefore, no dilution in the quality of the training results; the mother-resident's training is identical to that of the male residents in the department's traditional thirty-six-month program. All the requirements established for the residency program as a whole must be fulfilled, and residents are required to take the annual National Board of Medical Examiners' examination in psychiatry.

The resident salary of $5,640 a year is prorated for the women who are enrolled in the special program.

For mothers who have been retired from active participation in medicine due to their child-rearing responsibilities, the program provides tutorial instruction both in psychiatry and in other fields of medicine.

Weekly Seminars. A unique aspect of the New York Medical College program is the inclusion of a mandatory weekly seminar throughout the training period. This two-hour session "approximates a group psychotherapy experience and helps the physician-mothers resolve the inevitable conflicts deriving from their dual responsibility." [10]

"The girls themselves were sabotaging the program at first," Dr. Kaplan says. "They felt guilty, still felt they had to compete. This prompted the mothers' group therapy program—we had to remove this guilt about their contribution."

The resident-mothers have much in common, and they meet to

discuss their professional and personal problems and experiences. The group supervisor is a psychiatrist-mother and provides another factor usually lacking in conventional programs: an interested counselor to whom the residents can confidently turn for guidance and support. This psychiatrist has experienced the same problems the young mothers are now facing and solving.

Dr. Kaplan, who conducted these meetings initially, credits them with the success the program has achieved. "Such seminars are essential for any 'mother' program, especially at first. Irrational attitudes exist in the women themselves; they must recognize them and overcome them."

Another advantage accruing to these mother-residents is that they can take full advantage of the rich resources available at a good training institution. Formerly, no matter how hard a mother-doctor tried, the demands created by her dual role did not permit sufficient time to attend optional meetings, participate in individual investigation and research, or "become engaged in the intense interpersonal relationships which are a unique and important part of psychiatric training." [11]

A Positive Environment. Without sacrificing or diluting any of the requirements of good training, an atmosphere of flexibility has been created that is essential to the success of the program. Dr. Kaplan believes an environment where attention is paid to the individual's needs and problems is so important that without it such a program is doomed to failure.

Support must come from the directors of the educational program concerned, that is, hospital administrators, department chairmen, and faculty members. When such cooperation exists, "there is minimal irritation felt by male residents about the special arrangements made for their female counterparts." Fellow residents can be understanding of the two sets of demands made upon the mother-physician, and the positive environment permits the mother to take time off when necessary, to stay home with a sick child or cope with some other domestic emergency, without feeling guilt and hostility because she is away from the hospital.

"Our top management is very pro [the extended program]," Dr. Kaplan explains. "The lower management and other residents did not like the idea of the extended program at first. We talked with everyone concerned, told them this was it, we approved of it, and this was the way it would work. If anyone had any really serious objections and felt they could not work with the program, we told them they were free to leave. There was initial grumbling, and then it stopped."

Dr. Kaplan realizes that most people think they have good reasons for objecting to new ideas; those who object must be shown that they will be aided by the proposal, not hurt. In the case of the extended program, the mother-residents provide additional coverage in the department, rather than taking anything away from the regular residency program by their extended time schedules. The program does not threaten anyone, and this must be made clear to everyone involved.

The New York Medical College teaching staff has evaluated the clinical performance and academic knowledge of the resident-mothers and found both to compare favorably with those of the male residents.

"We have found that due to the resident-mothers' enthusiasm and maturity, their participation in the program has clearly been an asset and a cohesive force. In spite of certain scheduling modifications necessary for the mothers as a group, their presence has been in no way disruptive to our educational and service programs. There has been a surprising lack of absenteeism from their work, although it was made clear that the women could be excused for any reasonable domestic demand." [12]

This special program for mother-physicians has been approved by the American Board of Psychiatry. "In psychiatry there is great interest in attracting candidates for training who have satisfying personal lives and who are relatively free of debilitating emotional conflicts." [13] The attitude prevailing at NYMC is one that "recognizes and sympathetically accepts the occasional conflicts that may arise between home and professional role; it is believed that this attitude will diminish the guilt which is often experienced by women physicians who are mothers in their attempt to meet the exacting demands of both roles." [14]

Specialties Unsuited to Modified Time Schedules

Dr. Glen Leymaster, president of Woman's Medical College of Pennsylvania, is an advocate of flexible training schedules whenever possible. But he believes that not all specialties should have modified or extended time schedules.

"There are good reasons why some of the specialties will not permit part-time residency programs. Such fields as general surgery or obstetrics-gynecology demand full-time training. The experience of being on call for emergencies carries over from training into practice. The very best parts of the training come from prolonged experience with the very ill patients. This kind of responsibility cannot be acquired on a part-time basis."

In other words, the woman who intends to raise a family should select her specialty with care and thought for her combined goals.

Internship Programs

The internship remains one of the most inflexible obstacles to mother-doctors, who must complete this mandatory year of training in order to practice medicine and obtain licensing. The American Medical Association has changed the Essentials of an Approved Internship under Section IX to permit part-time internships "especially by women for whom full-time duties would not be possible because of family obligation." However, the *Directory of Approved Internships and Residencies* does not identify programs with part-time training arrangements.

Dr. Leymaster admits that he has been unsuccessful so far in arranging any modified time schedules for the woman interns in the hospitals affiliated with his college. His strongest recommendation is that women delay the arrival of children until the internship is completed.

Dr. Ruth Lawrence, in her study for the Macy conference, could not locate one internship that had been tailored to fit the needs of a mother-intern. Various mother-doctors, such as Lenor Zies (*see* Chapter 12), reported cooperation in working out equitable intern schedules during pregnancy, but such arrangements were made on an individual basis, after the woman took the initiative in requesting the arrangement. No general program or policy has been instituted, even in hospitals cooperating in the individual modified internships. Special arrangements in both internship and residency programs are not encouraged or sought by department heads, but are merely agreed to because of the need of the participant herself.

Cleveland's Pilot Program for Extended Internship and Residency. One pilot undertaking is just being established at the University Hospitals of Cleveland to attract young women who may be considering leaving the profession after medical school graduation. Two recent graduates, both young mothers, are sharing a part-time internship and residency program with extended schedules. They will take forty-eight months to complete a pediatric internship and a two-year residency, dividing a seventy-five-hour week of five working days plus two nights on call.

The training is as rigorous as in any conventional program, and the total time required for completion is not reduced but lengthened. The two mother-physicians take their night duty in two-month blocks to allow for unbroken time at home when they are not on duty. Salaries for doctors on the part-time and extended schedules are reduced to allow for the time adjustment, but over the total training period are equal to those of other house officers.

The reduced schedules are being offered in residency programs in other departments in the hospital, permitting a mother to reduce her schedule by half or one-third in order to be at home when her school-age children are. This stretches a regular two-year residency to four years in the former case. An alternative schedule allows mothers with older children to work full-time during the school year, but take summers and holidays off. Allowances are also made for special emergencies at home.

If the extended time or shared internship pilot program is successful, it can not only keep more mother-physicians active, but will also help to solve staffing problems at many hospitals with shortages of medical personnel.

Part-Time Internship Programs. The *Directory of Approved Internships and Residencies* now sanctions part-time internships "in the case of female graduates of medical schools who have obligations, especially to those of dependent children, which prevent them from engaging in full-time internship activities." [15]

"The Council [on Medical Education of the American Medical Association] does not wish to discourage the appointment of qualified female physicians to part-time internships, provided the responsible program director is able to arrange a program which meets the educational needs of the trainee and provided its total extent results in the sum of clinical experience and responsibilities acquired by an intern on a normal schedule."

What Remains to Be Done. A lot of groundwork must still be done to remove the stigma against part-time and extended internships and residencies so that more women will utilize such programs when they are offered. Carol Lopate has found that many women were reluctant to take advantage of such programs even when hospitals offered them,[16] and were still trying to be the equals of their male peers rather than differentiating themselves on the basis of family responsibilities. Dr. Kaplan's experiences were similar at the outset of the New York Medical College's mother-residents program. Woman interns and residents generally think they should keep their family life and problems to themselves, rather than admitting they have a justifiable reason for modified training programs. Mother medics are still on the defensive, trying to prove they can pull off two jobs to the men's one.

We need a universal concession to the demands in time and physical well-being made on the intern and resident. As the pressure eases and more sensible schedules become a reality for both men and women, the pressure on women to keep up with the men will lessen. In the long run, our country will benefit by the participation of more qualified physicians in the final stage of medical training.

Instead of permitting internships and residencies to go unfilled, or to be filled by foreign medical school graduates, we will be extending the opportunity to those who drop out of medicine because they cannot reconcile the demands of hospital training schedules with the requirements of family life.

"Plans should be made for decreasing the number of women who will be forced into retirement by the inappropriateness of their training or failure to anticipate the problems of combining career and child raising. It is here that we need to take a long look at our present situation." [17] We must constantly seek new programs that will provide a realistic means for women to complete their training while fulfilling their natural role as wife and mother. Sensible modifications in the internship and residency training of mother-doctors will alleviate the problem of "doctor dropouts" and the physician shortage in a more realistic manner than searching for medical Brunhildes.

Notes to Chapter Seventeen

1. John Z. Bowers, M.D., "Women in Medicine: An International Study," *New England Journal of Medicine,* 275: 362–365; August 18, 1966.
2. *Report for the Year 1966,* Josiah Macy, Jr., Foundation, New York, N.Y., 1966.
3. *Report for the Year 1967,* Josiah Macy, Jr., Foundation, New York, N.Y., 1967.
4. *Ibid.*
5. *Ibid.*
6. *Ibid.*
7. *Ibid.*
8. Harold I. Kaplan, M.D., Helen S. Kaplan, M.D., Ph.D., and Alfred M.

Freedman, M.D., "Psychiatric Residency Training Program for Physician Mothers: A Progress Report," *Journal of the American Medical Women's Association,* Vol. 19, No. 4, April, 1964. Pp. 285–289. Reprinted by permission.
9. *Ibid.*
10. *Ibid.*
11. *Ibid.*
12. *Ibid.*
13. Helen Singer Kaplan, M.D., Ph.D., "A New Concept of Graduate Training for Women Physicians," *Journal of the American Medical Women's Association,* Vol. 17, No. 10, October, 1962. Pp. 820–821. Reprinted by permission.
14. *Ibid.*
15. *Directory of Approved Internships and Residencies,* American Medical Association, 1966. P. 125.
16. Carol Lopate, *Women in Medicine,* Johns Hopkins Press, 1968. Pp. 115–116.
17. Ruth Anderson Lawrence, M.D., "The Training of Women Physicians," presented at Josiah Macy, Jr., Foundation conference on *Women for Medicine,* Dedham, Mass., October, 1966.

Chapter Eighteen

CONTINUING EDUCATION
OF THE WOMAN PHYSICIAN

"The better and more complete the training after graduation, the easier it is to obtain a job compatible with raising a family and the easier it is to stay with medicine instead of becoming a dropout. The information explosion in all scientific fields is tremendous, and in medicine it is beyond comprehension. A medical education is obsolete in five years unless it is constantly revitalized. While planning to mobilize the inactive woman physicians, plans must be made for decreasing the number of women who will be forced into retirement by the inappropriateness of their training or failure to anticipate the problems of combining career and child raising." [1]

The previous chapter outlined programs that enable women to continue their postgraduate training while beginning their families. This chapter will explore several pilot programs initiated to repair the technical obsolescence that quickly results when a woman leaves the profession to bear children and cannot find a way to return on a modified schedule. If she has not completed the internship, she will find very little opportunity to use her medical education. If many years have elapsed, much of her training will be obsolete. Retraining programs must have a great deal of flexibility to meet the needs of individuals reentering the profession after varying lengths of retirement.

It is hoped that the trend toward greater flexibility in internship and residency programs will produce a generation of woman physicians who can take advantage of continuing education courses and extended postgraduate training so that the more expensive retraining will not be as necessary. However, to meet today's critical physician shortage in this country, mobilization of women already possessing the M.D. can add a great many members to the medical profession in a short time. At best, this is a stopgap measure, but it salvages the investment society has already made in these women.

The two-day conference on Meeting Medical Manpower Needs: The Fuller Utilization of the Woman Physician, held in Washington, D. C., in January, 1968, pointed out that there were then about 1,800 physicians in the U.S. who were not in practice, of which 90 percent were women. About six hundred of them wanted to get back into practice if they could find refresher courses.[2] If the skills of these women could be mobilized, their contribution would exceed that of the graduating classes of half a dozen medical schools.

In her study of woman graduates of the University of Rochester School of Medicine, Dr. Ruth Lawrence found that "most women who were inactive expressed a desire to get back to medicine and asked for help in doing so." However, she also found, after searching for special retraining programs throughout the country, that no effort to encourage this type of salvage program for the woman doctor had been launched nationally.

Pacific Medical Center Retraining Program. The United States Public Health Service has awarded a grant to the continuing education department at Presbyterian Hospital of Pacific Medical Center in San Francisco for the benefit of inactive physicians desiring to complete residencies or update their professional knowledge. First priority is given to those who have been out of medical school for ten years or more, particularly those who are board-eligible, according to the center's announcement of the program.

The center has prepared a model of an ideal retraining program, with modifications applicable to general teaching hospitals, for the Public Health Service. The emphasis is on flexibility to fit individual needs, rather than on a highly structured training. "We hope this can then be used for programs which in the future may be funded from private or public sources," states Dr. Margaret Brown, the curriculum coordinator.[3]

The pilot program was established in September, 1966. The minimum time for retraining is six months, and the maximum one year.

Those who are not at the board-eligible level are offered a program of rotation through medicine, pediatrics, office gynecology, minor surgery, and emergency work. The training is full time.

In addition to classwork and lectures, the physicians go on hospital rounds. Much of the retraining takes place in clinical situations. The first months of instruction are devoted to a concentrated review of the basic medical subjects, with particular emphasis on the systems of the body. The aim is to enable the physicians to begin direct patient care as soon as possible.

Although the original aim of this program was to "retrain inactive woman physicians and return them to work," it was later modified to include men. Two male dropouts thus far have availed themselves of the intensified instruction.

In the twenty-six months (three of which are projected) that the program has been in operation at the time of writing, seventeen women and two men have taken part for periods of from four weeks to fourteen months. Three were graduates of foreign medical schools without licensure in the United States. They ranged in age from thirty to sixty-three years; their length of time away from practice ran from five to twenty-two years.

Their stipends follow Public Health Service fellowship rules: each fellow receives five thousand dollars per year as basic payment and five hundred dollars for each year of postdoctoral training (internship, residency, fellowship). According to the accepted Internal Revenue ruling, $3,600 of this is tax-exempt.

The actual cost of training one person is estimated at $548 per month, or $6,576 per year.[4] This sum includes the stipend or expense allowance for the trainee, except when he is in active practice.

"The low overhead," Dr. Brown points out, "was possible only because of the kindness of the staff and clinical faculty who gave so generously of their time in teaching."[5]

Dr. Brown's most recent report on the nineteen trainees stated that nine were employed or were continuing in formal residency training, three who had been on leave from active practice had returned, five were in training, the plans of one were incomplete, and one was seeking employment.

Dr. Brown evaluates the program as successful: "We consider retraining of inactive physicians as well as updating practicing physicians feasible and necessary. We consider the study successful and from it have prepared a model of what we would consider an ideal program as well as modifications for training in general medical teaching centers." [6]

Woman's Medical College Continuing Education Program. For many years, Woman's Medical College of Pennsylvania has been informally retraining woman physicians who had left active practice to raise families and then decided to return. In September, 1968, the college inaugurated its first formal program in continuing education, enrolling eight female physicians, all of whom had been out of the profession for five or more years. The general aim of the course, which lasts one academic year, is to update their medical knowledge and return these women to active practice.

A highly individualized approach is being used. Each doctor must describe her personal goal and then work toward it. There is little classroom training, and what there is takes place in small groups. The program is handled like a preceptorship for each participant. Because so much of the training is on a one-to-one basis with faculty members, Dr. Glen Leymaster estimates that the annual cost for retraining one woman is about nine thousand to ten thousand dollars.

Dr. Leymaster justifies so expensive a venture for two reasons. First, the investment has already been made in the woman's education, and her talents and training will lie fallow without this updating. Second, she can be ready to practice at the end of a year of intensified study, if this is her objective, although some women want to pursue specialty training.

"These women are the ones who want to provide patient care; this program is not designed for the individual who is going into a research career. Therefore, we feel it is an important step in providing physicians who are so urgently needed in as short a time as possible," Dr. Leymaster says.

Dr. Leymaster notes the importance of self-confidence in any physician's ability to function to the best of his potential. He states that several women in the program would be perfectly competent to go into a residency but need the year to give them self-confidence. He believes that once they have updated their skills and familiarized themselves with new developments in the profession, at least one or two will go directly into their residencies on a full-time basis.

Dr. Leymaster plans to retrain ten to twelve doctor dropouts in the Woman's Medical College program each year. His greatest obstacle to date has been lack of the funds required for so expensive a project, yet one so urgently needed by society. The program is in part supported by a Macy Foundation grant of thirty thousand dollars.

Although Woman's Medical College only recently began seeking such aid, and some promised funds have been withdrawn, "I think we can do better," Dr. Leymaster says. He believes it is the responsibility of everyone in the profession to spell out the need more effectively.

"But our continuing education program will continue," Dr. Leymaster emphasizes.

Informal Retraining. The pediatric department of the University of Rochester (New York) School of Medicine has taken positive steps to encourage the dropout woman doctor to return to the fold. Mother-physicians can spend a few hours a week sitting in on classes, can see patients at the large teaching hospital affiliated with the medical school, or can "just kibitz." There is an open-door policy at "grand rounds," and the women are welcome to attend whenever convenient. In addition, a part-time associate residency program has been arranged for women who have been away from medicine for between five and twenty years; the program enables them to resume their training and refresh their knowledge of medicine in general.

More programs of this nature are needed throughout the nation, particularly in areas inaccessible to the large metropolitan medical centers. Women who are active in medicine can do a great deal to help bring about the changes that will help their fellow doctors return to practice. Such programs must be carefully planned, however, particularly when they are arranged on an individual basis and are not patterned after a model as part of general administrative policy. In addition, care must be taken to insure that the training provided in the program is equal in every respect to the training offered in the regular full-time residency as required by the particular specialty board.

Dr. Ruth Lawrence recently completed a follow-up study of several retired women in the Rochester community who had returned to complete their training in experimental modified-time programs. Her findings point up the obstacles to be overcome before such programs can be successful and acceptable in the everyday realm of medical education and postgraduate training:

One woman—whose four children had already grown—returned to a part-time residency shared with two other girls, after a twenty-year gap. She found she was putting in full-time hours but receiving part-time credit (and pay). She decided to take a full-time appointment and complete her requirements. She has just completed her Board requirements and accepted a staff appointment in a community medical project.

A second—whose four children were in high school, ages 13 to 18—found she too was putting in full-time hours for part-time credit and pay. She too has decided to try a year on a full-time appointment, which will complete her requirements. She had been retired 18 years.

A third—who just gave birth to her third child and had been out of medicine only five years—found clinical pediatrics incompatible with her young family. She has taken a residency in pathology where the program has been ideally tailored to her needs, even to having the summer off to be with her children.

A fourth woman, with four school-age children, took a part-time residency in psychiatry theoretically styled after the New York Medical College program. She quickly found it was not part-time. She found as the only part-time person working within a residency structured for full time that she was quickly involved as much as the others—again getting only part-time credit and pay. She has discontinued her training until her children are grown. She has taken a part-time job with a Family Practice Program.[7]

Unless the schedule is carefully designed and maintained, part-time work often eases into a full-time commitment. For this reason, the New York Medical College's extended residency in psychiatry has been successful, while the program of institutions that copied only some of New York's arrangements have not. Once a mother has taken the time to get dressed, make baby-sitting arrangements, and commute to the job location, she may as well put in a full day's work, as she will have little time to accomplish anything at home.

In Rochester, Dr. Lawrence has been directing her efforts to tutoring individuals in various stages of their schooling and talking to many woman candidates for admission to medical school or residency programs. She is doing on a personal basis what should be a general practice in all medical school counseling. Many women now in medicine could imitate her by trying to help girls just entering the profession. If enough woman doctors would contribute, they might initiate a whole tradition of counseling those who are to follow them.

"I have been consistently impressed with the number of girls who plan to marry, have children, and carry on—but have not considered in practical fashion what this might entail or what particular specialties might be most easily pursued," Dr. Lawrence comments.

Girls, ask the woman who's been there.

Mother-medics, give the next generation a few minutes of your time and some practical suggestions.

Notes to Chapter Eighteen

1. Ruth Anderson Lawrence, M.D., "The Training of Women Physicians," presented at the Josiah Macy, Jr., Foundation conference on *Women for Medicine,* Dedham, Mass., October, 1966.
2. Personal communication from Albert M. Betcher, M.D., of the American Society of Anesthesiologists, delegate to the conference on Meeting Medical Manpower Needs, August 13, 1968.
3. Personal communication from Margaret L. Brown, M.D., Curriculum Coordinator, Physicians' Trainee Program, Pacific Medical Center, July 5, 1968.
4. Personal communication from Margaret L. Brown, M.D., September 5, 1968.
5. *Ibid.*
6. *Ibid.*
7. Personal communication from Ruth A. Lawrence, M.D., Assistant Professor of Pediatrics, University of Rochester School of Medicine, August 16, 1968.

Chapter Nineteen

THE CHALLENGE AHEAD

The National Institutes of Health have just published the results of a study to isolate the obstacles keeping women from graduate study, with particular emphasis on the health and science fields. The study also sought to identify the factors that would influence more women to complete graduate training. The findings of this *Special Report on Women and Graduate Study* substantiate the long-standing impression that the major obstacles to graduate study by women are: (1) financial barriers and (2) family responsibilities. To overcome these obstacles, it will be necessary to provide competently staffed, conveniently located child-care centers and greatly increased opportunities to complete training on a part-time basis.[1]

The study also revealed that repeated graduate enrollment was twice as likely for the woman who received a stipend as for one who did not. Therefore, an increased number of stipends would obviously induce more women to enter the fields of science and medicine.

Eight out of ten women still feel that becoming a physician is too demanding to combine with family responsibilities, and approximately half feel that women cannot pursue this profession on a part-time basis.[2] As illustrated by the programs and case histories described throughout this book, that simply is no longer the case. Medicine is a satisfying and stimulating career to which women can and should aspire.

In the three-year period following college graduation that was covered in the NIH study, the greatest net loss of women from their planned career fields was in areas of prime importance to medical research and education. The net loss to medicine was 48 percent of the girls who as college seniors intended to pursue this career.[3]

Recent changes are encouraging. The American Medical Association now sanctions part-time internships and residencies, and many of the specialty boards approve part-time residency training and extended programs. These programs will benefit women who want to combine career and family, provided they can locate such programs and are able to take advantage of them. The deadlock has been broken, however. More and more part-time opportunities are being established, and recent findings support the view that more women would continue to participate in medicine for the greater part of their lives if they could practice part-time. The hard statistics and results revealed by this enlightening study cannot be denied. It is now up to both the medical community and the women in medicine to press for needed reforms as quickly as possible.

The following suggestions on what needs to be done are intended to alert young women just entering the profession to areas where their interest and influence can effect change. It is a temptation in all academic areas today to perpetuate existing situations because consciously or unconsciously, one wants others to suffer just as he has suffered. If we recognize this "emotional investment" (as one psychiatrist called it) and look at medical training rationally, we can select the portions that actually prepare a doctor and discard those that merely serve as hazing.

Counseling

When women are aware of the problems involved in the dual roles of medicine and child raising, they can plan realistically how to deal with conflicts that otherwise might cause them to drop out of active practice. Many mother-physicians admitted they had not known what it entailed to raise a family and remain medically active, and had felt guilty when they found they could not do so much in either role as was expected of them. Women should search out information on every career in medicine that offers them working hours and responsibilities compatible with family life. Advice on appropriate career choices and training plans must be available early to be most effective, and proper counseling can provide it. But counseling must be more than assisting a student in filling out forms. It should aid a girl in deciding how best to make her own special contribution to medicine.

At the high school and undergraduate college level, more informed counseling of the potential female medical student is needed. Girls should be encouraged to prepare themselves academically in the sciences and mathematics beginning in the early years of high school. Medical schools can help by inviting high school counselors to their campuses for briefings and tours of the educational facilities.

All too often, a girl is discouraged early in her schooling and told that women do not have a chance in medicine. As was pointed out in earlier chapters, women are accepted into medical schools at almost the same rate as men, even under today's limited and highly competitive selection system.

In many high schools and colleges, members of the science faculty also serve as premedical advisers. These teachers usually are not particularly interested in recruiting, or even encouraging, students for medicine. They are more likely to persuade their most talented students to pursue careers in the physical sciences and to tell girls that they do not have a chance for acceptance into medical school. In other words, much of the prejudice against women operates before they even apply to medical school, and only the hardiest and most determined candidates survive to make application. The promotion of the physical sciences is not altogether unjustified. Greater amounts of financial aid have been available in the physical sciences in recent decades, and the student in need of money is often steered away from medicine and into another field for this reason. Students who do not meet the academic requirements are also well-advised to seek less demanding areas of study.

The majority of successful medical school applicants, of course, come from high schools with an atmosphere of intellectual excellence and strong science departments. Even with a minimum of good guidance counseling, a student whose interest is stimulated by exposure to informative talks and field trips can be motivated to prepare for a medical career. If girls would only take advantage of the right curriculum, they would strengthen their background from the beginning and increase their chances for acceptance.

John H. Wulsin, M.D., of the University of Cincinnati College of Medicine, writes:

We must get the true message to the science teachers and counselors particularly at the high school level; that is, to encourage the capable girls to go to college with good science facilities, to take the required courses for medical school, and then finally to make the decision about applying during their junior year in college. The premed advisers in college must be told by the medical schools that girls are sought for and are accepted in the same proportions as boys, and these advisers must be pleaded with not to dissuade the motivated, capable female from applying.[4]

Surprisingly, one of the most critical needs for counseling of women exists in the medical schools themselves. A female adviser could offer continuity of advice and support to female students throughout their four years of medical education. In the clinical years particularly, students are rotated so quickly through the services that they do not have much chance to establish rapport with individual faculty members and feel they have no one to turn to for advice or constructive suggestions.

Young married women approaching the demanding year of internship feel intense guilt at the number of hours they must be away from their families. Group therapy and similar approaches allow them to meet and share their common problems. Realistic attitudes on the part of school administrators, department chairmen, and chiefs of service can help diminish the guilt that is often experienced by women attempting to meet the exacting demands of their dual roles.

Women should be told while in medical school that the more training they complete, the easier it will be to find jobs in medicine with predictable hours. "For those women about to be graduated, a program of counseling directed at the special problems of the woman doctor should be made available in all medical schools."[5] Women already on medical faculties have a responsibility to share their knowledge and experience with the young women coming into the field.

Dr. Glen Leymaster, president of Woman's Medical College of Pennsylvania, believes it is the duty of every girl considering a medical career to learn everything she can about the profession and to seek advice. "The important problems are her own," he points out. "If she wants marriage and children, she must plan for the problems of competition from these demands with her need for continuing education. She needs counseling at every stage of her preparation."

Dr. Leymaster recommends that girls seek out and talk to a number of woman physicians with a variety of professional experience. The advice a girl follows will depend upon which career pattern she has in mind. "A girl should especially confer with the women who have become the kind of physician she wants to be."

"A girl should do some very careful thinking about her future ten years hence," Dr. Leymaster concludes. "She is doing a disservice to everyone to assume she can do it as a man could."

Application Procedures

The overlapping of applications to medical schools creates an unnecessary complication and often causes delays in acceptance. The current average is four applications for each student, but many apply to a dozen or more schools. The time, expense, and clerical work involved justifies a new look at our medical school application system.

Several schools have put into effect an early acceptance plan that postpones the submission and processing of the detailed supporting data that must accompany every application form until the candidate has been tentatively accepted. A preliminary application form allows for the early screening out of obviously unqualified applicants, who, while still in their senior year of college, can then begin to prepare for alternate careers. Under the early acceptance plan, the student applies initially only to his first choice in a medical school, with the understanding that he will receive an early decision on his application. If refused, he can request admission to other medical schools, or he can change his career plans and move into an allied field. Academic medicine is one possibility open to such a student with a graduate degree in one of the medical or physical sciences. If not academically qualified, the student may decide on a paramedical profession.

This approach could alleviate the problem of a great surplus of applications at the handful of prestige schools while lesser-known schools have seats available.

One dean of admissions does not see much possibility of increased efficiency unless the present application system is completely revised. He suggests that a national system would be a great improvement. He cites the example of Italy, where a student does not apply to a particular school but to a "medical school in Italy," expressing a preference. "Then one gets assigned," the dean affirms.

The selection of applicants also could benefit from a new approach. Rather than trying to choose a certain kind of student who will not drop out of the current curriculum, conventional medical training could be modified so that a greater variety of personality types, both men and women, could participate. The medical school itself can be a source of attrition, and medical educators are just becoming aware of this. The schools tend to choose an independent type of person, and then offer a curriculum that stifles creativity and discourages independence. The growing trend toward increased flexibility in premedical background and medical school studies should permit more students to qualify than ever before. This is a positive approach toward increasing the number of physicians.

Housing

Fifty-six percent of woman medical students marry doctors while they are in medical school.[6] These couples have great difficulty in finding suitable places to live. In the majority of cases, dormitories are provided only for single students, and there has been little realistic planning for the increasing number of married couples in student bodies throughout the country. The provision of housing facilities near the school or hospital would relieve one of the conditions that force women to drop out of medicine for nonacademic reasons. A nursery school, a laundry, and cheerful apartments could be incorporated into the institution's physical facilities and would help to attract and keep talented people.

"University regulations which do not permit the use of university housing if the husband is not studying or working in the university discriminate against women in the health field." [7] One of the recommendations resulting from the conference on Fuller Utilization of the Woman Physician is that "medical schools (independent or in a university complex) revise their housing policies to permit on-campus or university residence for families of married women students, to provide adequate day care for children, to make available suitable dwellings near the medical school." [8] The profession must recognize that married medical students, both men and women, are no longer rare, and the need for better housing and living conditions is increasing. At present, most university bulletins merely tell students who desire married couples' quarters to put their names on a waiting list—in other words, there hasn't been any housing available for you around here for a long time, and there won't be in the foreseeable future!

Child Care

Dr. Helen Kaplan, a psychiatrist and mother, describes the most critical need for the woman who plans to practice medicine while raising a family:

"The whole thing rests on the availability of child care. If you don't have it, you cannot take advantage of any program, no matter how well designed. It has been demonstrated that substitute mother care does not hurt the children at all.

"I do not favor group care before three years of age; until they reach this age, children should be cared for at home. Therefore, tax deductions for household help and child care are a must. If a man can deduct for his secretary, a woman should be able to deduct for her required help."

For children over three, both preschoolers and youngsters who require only after-school care, provision must be made for more child-care centers. This is a common need of all working and professional women, but the extent of the shortage becomes glaringly apparent when woman doctors, at the top of the nation's pay scale, are unable to secure suitable help.

Hospitals and medical centers can render a dual service to members in the health professions by establishing day nurseries, nursery schools, and kindergartens, with intelligent supervisory personnel, where physician-mothers can leave their children with the assurance that they are not being neglectful. Dr. John Bowers, president of the Macy Foundation, suggests that metropolitan centers with a number of medical schools, hospitals, library facilities, and training programs initiate cooperative efforts encompassing integrated course work, internships, and residencies. These centers could be adapted to the needs of young women with domestic responsibilities by providing child-care facilities for personnel.[9]

One hospital director commented that his institution had established a day nursery, hoping to lure more qualified woman physicians into service, but that the nursery was utilized mainly by the paramedical personnel; most of the mother-physicians did not use it. While it may be that mother-physicians prefer to have their children cared for in their own homes, this is no excuse for deferring the establishment of a child-care center for hospital personnel.

The doctor, because of her longer training and higher earning ability, should have the option of providing whatever care she believes is best for her children. Even if she chooses home care, when a nursemaid or governess fails to report for work or quits without notice the mother should have a workable alternative, such as the use of institutional day-care facilities, while she seeks a replacement. Such facilities—simply by being there—provide the peace of mind necessary for a woman to continue in a professional position of great responsibility. A woman would not have the guilt feelings that often lead to dropping out if she always had available a well-run nursery instead of having to rely on makeshift baby-sitting arrangements in emergencies.

The Women's Bureau of the U. S. Department of Labor has been participating actively in efforts to encourage the expansion of child-care services for all working mothers. Former Director Mary Keyserling reports that "in view of the present urgent need for hospital workers, we are now conducting a survey of child-care centers established by hospitals for the children of hospital personnel . . . we have already learned of a number of new centers and have received expressions of interest from hospitals who do not as yet have such facilities." [10] Mother-physicians can take an active part in helping to establish such facilities in their areas.

Programs under the Manpower Development Training Act and similar legislation currently are undertaking to train women for work in child-care centers. Federal funds are being allotted for the development of day-care projects and training programs to improve the qualifications and performance of workers. The Women's Bureau has been participating in these efforts and in the preparation of recommended codes of standards for household employees and employers.

These federally supported programs are scattered throughout the country. In addition, both private and community agencies are working in the field. In Denver, for example, the Colorado Department of Employment is conducting classes for household employees, upgrading their basic education and providing them with counseling and placement service. Similar programs are springing up everywhere; the local office of your state employment agency can tell you if there is one in your area.

A 1965 study by the American Medical Association, the Association of American Medical Colleges, and the American Medical Women's Association reported on the professional characteristics of male and female physicians who had graduated from medical school during the period 1931 through 1956. The major focus of the study was on the practice patterns of woman physicians, and the findings underscored the importance of the availability of child care.

Data obtained in the study indicated a trend toward earlier marriage by medical students and physicians in training. Almost 30 percent of the woman physicians had married by the time of graduation from medical school, twice the percentage of an earlier study that included data on woman medical graduates of 1925 to 1940.[11]

The figures also showed a trend toward the establishment of families during the years of medical education: "It is thus apparent that the proportions of woman physicians marrying and bearing children during the years of their medical education and subsequent training have shown a rapid rate of increase and that these factors must be strongly considered in relation to the effect they have on potential professional activity of women medical graduates." [12]

Just how strong the effect had become was illustrated when the full- and part-time categories of the 1964 professional activity of woman physicians were compared on the basis of marital status and number of children. "Married women with three or more children constitute the only active group reporting a slightly smaller proportion engaged in full-time activity than are engaged in part-time activity. Reports of no professional activity range from 2.8% of single women to 17.6% of married women with three or more children." The study established an inverse relationship between the number of children and professional activity, although the two were not mutually exclusive. Large numbers of married women with several children were still actively pursuing professional careers. It would seem that child-care availability was a critical factor, as the women who had curtailed their professional activity at some time during their careers reported family responsibility as the primary reason.[13]

Tax Incentives
The President's Commission on the Status of Women examined the question of tax deductions for child-care expenses. Its recommendations, published in 1963, were as follows:

"Tax deductions for child care expenses of working mothers should be kept commensurate with the median income of couples when both husband and wife are engaged in substantial employment. The present limitation on their joint income, above which deductions are not allowable, should be raised. Additional deductions, of lesser amounts, should be allowed for children beyond the first. The 11-year age limit for child care deductions should be raised." [14]

The report states that, while the advantage from any allowable tax deduction still accrues to some moderate-income and to low-income families . . . the limit above which deductions are not allowed has become unrealistic. . . . The majority of working couples are therefore ineligible for deductions . . . moreover, no account has been taken of the number of children that must be cared for." [15]

While the 1964 Revenue Act did liberalize the tax allowance to some extent, the Women's Bureau agrees that the deduction as it presently stands does not offer much relief to the professional woman who wishes to work and must have assistance in running her home. For many woman doctors with small children, active practice has become an expensive hobby. Various bills have been introduced in Congress that would eliminate the income ceiling and/or the dollar limit on the child-care deduction.

In the April 1968 Report on the Task Force on Social Insurance and Taxes to the Citizens' Advisory Council on the Status of Women, another approach to the needs of working mothers was offered. The Task Force felt that regardless of the extent of the deduction allowed, it would be ineffective in making child care services available to any very large number of working wives, since most such wives are members of the families that cannot afford to pay for such services. The Task Force recommended that the tax provisions be phased out and that immediate steps be taken to expand child care services so that they would be available to persons in all income levels, with charges based on ability to pay. However, it should be noted that the Citizens' Advisory Council continues to support the Federal income tax deduction for child care.[16]

This development is important to all professional women, since doing away with the tax provisions in favor of expanded child-care services would eliminate the option of providing child care in the home without financial penalty. The need is great throughout the country for more child-care facilities, and professional women should make their feelings in the matter known, through letters to their congressmen and local political action. Women must take a more active interest in legislation that so personally affects their homes, their careers, and their freedom to choose without penalty the type of domestic service that best suits the needs of their families.

The American Medical Women's Association is on record in favor of retaining tax deductions, but increasing them to a more realistic level. The association recognizes that the need is more complex than for simple baby-sitting:

> In discussing tax deductions for household help . . . it was noted that child care is really only one facet of the homemaker's task. Homemaking is the job of creating a climate for personal fulfillment for oneself and others. It is both an art and a complex managerial task. . . . Women do not buy full-time homemaker service with a marriage license, but must pay with time and muscle, or with hard cash. The complexity of the job increases with the number of people in the household.
>
> The Congress of the United States is obviously unaware of this problem. So are business leaders, heads of University Departments, and quite a few husbands. Yet the reality faces all 18,000 women physicians and untold thousands of other career women every day.[17]

The AMWA is fully aware that one of the greatest handicaps a woman physician faces when she tries to remain active while raising a family is the lack of reliable and competent domestic help.

The Women's Auxiliary of the American Medical Association is considering expansion of its homemaker services program, with the needs of woman physicians particularly in mind. Such professional organizations, plus the federal agencies concerned with medical manpower on the one hand and career development for the disadvantaged on the other, offer avenues of action leading to solutions of the child-care problem and household-help shortage. The active participation in such endeavors of young women entering the medical profession will increase the chances of success.

Professional Organizations
In spite of the fact that a number of national conferences have recommended legislative action regarding tax deductions for child

care and household help, among other needs, very little can be seen in the way of results. Medical women can work toward these goals through existing organizations, such as the American Medical Women's Association.

It should not be expected that medical organizations composed primarily of male members will voluntarily devote much time to strictly feminine projects. However, their support can be gained by stressing the relationship between the women's needs and the effect of legislative inaction on female practice rates. Both the American Medical Association and the Association of American Medical Colleges have expressed concern about the practice rates of woman physicians, and they are directly affected by the continuance of a situation that contributes to the dropout rate. The congressional torpor on the proposed changes in tax deductions could be changed through effective lobbying and by making the tax matter a campaign issue.

On projects such as this, woman doctors should join with other organizations of professional women who have the same needs. Business and professional women's clubs, professional fraternities and sororities, civic clubs, and university women's groups can be utilized to formulate policy and work for action.

Too much time has elapsed since the recommendations of the President's Commission were first published in 1963. The needs of mother-professionals must be met, and women must organize more effectively to get favorable legislation if they are to participate to their fullest potential in their chosen careers.

Financial Aid

A community that has a physician shortage—and there are few in our country today that do not—can take positive steps to increase both the quantity and the quality of the health care available to its citizens. Any community can provide appropriate training programs in its local hospitals for qualified woman medics. Such projects should be supported by local organizations and could be administered by local medical societies.

The general public does not think of medicine as a profession that requires financial aid. Yet many students from middle- or low-income families are deterred from even attempting to obtain medical educations because of the large debts they would incur during their training. Families of limited means with both sons and daughters to educate will usually decide to invest their money in the sons;

the daughters often are discouraged, either directly or subtly, from seeking graduate study. Some medical school admissions officers admit privately that the candidate with financial backing is preferred over the equally well-qualified one who will have to accumulate large debts in order to complete school. Studies of the socioeconomic backgrounds of medical students bear out this observation; they show that, although the lower socioeconomic classes are well represented in state universities, a disproportionately small percentage are accepted into the medical schools.

Mary I. Bunting, president of Radcliffe College, sees federal assistance as the best answer to the financial problems of students, and adds a practical twist:

"Eventually, I hope that qualified men and women wishing to get medical training will be financed by the nation as a valuable national resource. If they have lucrative practices later, the government can collect sufficient income tax to more than cover the costs. In the meantime, I'd favor programs to assist individuals directly and traineeships to institutions." [18]

Women's clubs, service organizations, and local medical societies can support the qualified women in their localities and help them financially to complete their education. Funding at the critical point, when a woman physician begins her family and is in danger of dropping out of the profession because she cannot assume the added burden of child-care costs, would keep additional doctors active in the community.

"A community should realize the resources it can tap right in its own area," Dr. Ruth Lawrence explains. "A woman doctor with an established home and family is not going to leave the community. Whatever is invested in retraining a doctor who dropped out of practice is going to benefit the people who support her."

A woman with a home and children often cannot commute long distances, or even to a nearby large city, to take advantage of a formalized retraining program or part-time residency. For this reason, these programs should not be centralized but should be sprinkled across the country. There are many excellent community medical institutions that could train mother-physicians and retrain doctor dropouts.

Those who are planning or have established such projects recommend that the agencies funding them award their grants directly to individuals, rather than to a large institution or city agency. If the grant is in the form of a fellowship, the first thirty-six hundred dollars is tax-free, a big help to the woman who must pay a baby-sitter or household help. Some government grants are in the form of fellowships, for instance, Labor Department-sponsored retraining program at Pacific Medical Center (*see* Chapter 18).

"If the individual received the funds, any hospital, anywhere, could retrain retired women," Dr. Lawrence states. "A woman could first find out how much and what type of training she needed —exactly what she would require to resume active practice. She could then apply to the fund source, setting out her program as planned at an approved medical facility. Such programs would, of course, have to meet preestablished minimum standards."

A program of this sort could be administered by a regional hospital council serving a statewide or interstate area that included some metropolitan centers as well as small cities and towns. When grants are awarded on a regional basis, a woman who lives in a small town no more than one hundred miles from a major city can take advantage of training in her own place of residence without leaving her family. This method serves the majority of people concentrated in big cities without denying an equal opportunity to those scattered about the countryside. Often, a small city or town derives greater benefit from the addition of one practicing physician than a large city from half a dozen.

Support from the Medical Profession Itself

"The general trend in the proportion of women accepted by medical schools has shown a slight increase in recent years," Dr. Davis G. Johnson of the Association of American Medical Colleges reports.[19]

However, there is still prejudice against admitting women to medical school: "Women physicians complain that our medical schools have 'secret' quotas for women and adhere to them very strictly. Such quotas do exist in some institutions, but they are breaking down." This was a finding of the Macy Foundation, published in its annual report for 1967.[20] The number of women graduated from medical school has remained fairly constant over the last few decades, despite the greatly increased number being trained at the college level in recent years.

"We need to have more leading male members of our medical faculties and the medical profession informed about and interested in the opportunities for women in medicine and in helping them solve the problems that a woman medical student, or woman doctor, must face." [21]

The medical schools play an important role in recruiting talented students for medicine; little of their recruiting is directed toward the top female students. Increased communication is needed between the medical schools and the colleges. Many of the girls who walk off with the honors in high school and college could be successful medical students. Yet little is done to seek them out and attract them to medicine.

"The anti-feminists point out that we must educate two women to obtain time in medicine equal to that which we obtain from one man. Yet 90 per cent of women graduates report they are in part-time or full-time medical work." [22] Admissions committees often face strong opposition to women from some faculty members. The women themselves can do more to ease these attitudes by not trying to attempt the impossible, by dropping any vestigial suffragette attitudes of belligerence, and by completing whatever they undertake.

Keeping Commitments

A woman must consider first what is involved in any conflicting demands on her time, and then plan her training with a realistic approach to her goal. She must realize that once she has made a commitment, no matter how difficult it may be to complete, she must fulfill it.

The acceptance of a residency is essentially a contract. Department chairmen complain that, again and again, woman physicians make agreements to accept residencies, and then break them. The fact that a married woman must be able to move if her husband is transferred, and must subordinate her career plans to his, is recognized as a widespread problem. It can be resolved by realistic counseling and a sense of responsibility on the part of the woman herself.

Be honest about your situation when accepting any appointment, educators advise. If possible, get established in a permanent location before taking on an obligation such as a residency. One doctor gave an example of a young woman who had planned wisely around her family demands. Her husband, also a medical student, faced military duty after his graduation. She decided to graduate, too, complete her internship, and then join him on his overseas tour of duty. She had two children during the overseas period, because she believed it was a good time at which to interrupt her training. While overseas she could devote her full time to her husband and babies, and be ready on returning to the states to begin a full-time residency. This she has done, the doctor reported, and was in her last year of residency at the time of writing.

"There is a general feeling [among male administrators] that women believe they can accept a residency, and then, just before beginning, can bring up reasons which are particularly feminine for not keeping the commitment," admits Dr. Glen Leymaster, president of Woman's Medical College of Pennsylvania.

"Any department head who has been placed in the position of arguing against motherhood is hurt by the experience; he is not likely to appoint another female to a residency in his department," says Dr. Leymaster.

In any institution where such a reneging has occurred, the chances for acceptance are lessened for all the women who will follow. "The woman physician must lean over backward to keep her commitments, once they are made," Dr. Leymaster emphasizes.

Careful career planning, followed by a realistic acceptance of responsibility and a firm determination to fulfill her commitments, should be the aim of every young woman from medical school through the completion of her training.

Notes to Chapter Nineteen

1. "Special Report on Women and Graduate Study," National Institutes of Health, U.S. Department of Health, Education, and Welfare. *Resources for Medical Research,* Report No. 13, June, 1968. Pp. 3, 7, and 8 of "Selected Highlights."
2. *Ibid.*
3. *Ibid.*
4. John H. Wulsin, M.D., "Admission of Women to Medical School," *Journal of the American Medical Women's Association,* Vol. 21, No. 8, August, 1966. Pp. 674–676.
5. Ruth Anderson Lawrence, M.D., "The Training of Women Physicians," presented at Josiah Macy, Jr., Foundation conference on *Women for Medicine,* Dedham, Mass., October, 1966.
6. Leona Baumgartner, M.D., "The American Woman Physician: The Challenge of Fuller Utilization," from report of conference on Meeting Medical Manpower Needs: The Fuller Utilization of the Woman Physician, January 12–13, 1968, Washington D.C. Sponsored by American Medical Women's Association, President's Study Group on Careers for Women, Women's Bureau of U.S. Department of Labor. Published by

American Medical Women's Association, 1968. P. 15. Reprinted by permission.

7. George T. Harrell, M.D., "Highlights of Workshop III, The Postgraduate School Years," *op. cit.* P. 69.
8. "Recommendations," *op. cit.* P. 91.
9. John Z. Bowers, M.D., "Women in Medicine: An International Study," *New England Journal of Medicine,* 275: 362–365, August 18, 1966.
10. Personal communication from Mary Dublin Keyserling, Director, Women's Bureau, U.S. Department of Labor, September 30, 1968.
11. "Facts on Prospective and Practicing Women in Medicine," prepared for conference on Meeting Medical Manpower Needs: The Fuller Utilization of the Woman Physician, January 12–13, 1968.
12. *Ibid.*
13. *Ibid.*
14. *American Women,* report of the President's Commission on the Status of Women, Washington, D.C., 1963.
15. *Ibid.*
16. Keyserling, *op. cit.*
17. Elizabeth A. McGraw, M.D., "Tax Deductions," *Journal of the American Medical Women's Association,* August, 1967. P. 585. Reprinted by permission.
18. Personal communication from Mary I. Bunting, Ph.D., President, Radcliffe College, Cambridge, Mass., November 4, 1968.
19. *Journal of the American Medical Assosiation,* Vol. 198, No. 8, November 21, 1966. Figures and comparisons also made from the same study published in 1965: Davis G. Johnson, Ph.D., "The Study of Applicants, 1964–1965," *Journal of Medical Education,* Vol. 40, November, 1965.
20. *Report for the Year 1967,* Josiah Macy, Jr., Foundation, New York, N.Y., 1967.
21. *Ibid.*
22. *Ibid.*

Chapter Twenty

CONCLUSION

During the three years of research, travel, interviewing, writing, and revising that have gone into this book, many significant changes in medical education favorable to women, and to medical students in general, have taken place. At the outset of my inquiries, many questions brought negative responses. I asked questions such as: "Why couldn't medical education be shortened in some cases?" "Could some phases of training be scheduled part-time for women with families?" "Could overlapping courses in the basic sciences be combined?" The initial reactions of "We can't do that without sacrificing quality" gradually changed to "We are now in the process of revising our curriculum," or "So-and-so college has a program like that now." Instead of being eyed suspiciously as an iconoclast or suffragette, I began to share in enthusiastic discussions with modern medical educators who sincerely want to see the old order changed.

Americans are demanding to know why we are faced with an overwhelming physician shortage when we have such a great number of talented, college-trained youth. There is no valid reason for a country so rich in resources—human and fiscal—to deny modern health care to many of its citizens. Nothing can justify the neglect of talent in the feminine half of our population.

The stubborn refusal to educate sufficient physicians to meet the needs of our people has brought us to a grave crisis. The archaic attitude of our society toward women in medicine has denied us many qualified professionals who could alleviate the situation.

Recent conferences have shown the need for giving greater recognition to women who have been successful in medicine. I have done so liberally throughout this book by presenting the stories and opinions of many women who are successful doctors while also leading full and active lives as wives and mothers. It is my hope that they will serve as models to girls just entering medicine.

Realizing that "success" is more than achievement in a single area, I have tried to show that a woman does not have to relinquish her femininity to be a successful doctor. To be satisfying and rewarding, her life must be the sum of all her activities. She need not sacrifice her desire for marriage and children, nor feel guilty about tending to these obligations in addition to those of a physician.

The choice of satisfied and well-adjusted professional women as models in this book was deliberate, and not intended to be misleading. The aim was to show some of the many possible combinations of career and home that *do* work, and to reveal the attitudes and values that lead to positive adjustments in the face of various conflicts. When I told the story of a busy mother-intern who has full-time help in her home, I hoped to imply that not having such help would be an additional hardship. This is one of the considerations that each woman interested in medicine must take into account before deciding whether she could cope with the dual responsibilities.

Nor do I wish to recruit women who are unsuited to medicine as a career, or to encourage unqualified girls to attempt the impossible. However, for the girl who is uncertain but has an absorbing interest in medicine and science, a premedical education will never be wasted. Many related careers are just beginning to open up—the physician's assistant is one—in addition to the traditional paramedical professions. The demand for health care personnel will far outstrip the supply for decades to come. A girl with a sound academic background in the medical sciences will always find herself sought after. If you aspire to medicine and think you can make it, give yourself every advantage in the way of preparation. Should you not be accepted to medical school, you will still have an invaluable education that is well suited to many other richly rewarding careers.

Our society has wasted much valuable feminine talent that it urgently needs. We must change our entire attitude toward gifted women, and prepare them from their earliest years to make a contribution.

Most women do not—and should not—want to compete with men on male grounds. One of the most important things a woman has to offer any profession is her femininity. We need more than a greater quantity of doctors. We need the *qualities* that only women can bring to medicine.

INDEX

INDEX

for Negro students, 97–100, 103–104, 108
postgraduate, 107–108
scholarships, 95–98, 100–101, 104
local funds, 104
medical school, 100
undergraduate, 95–98
undergraduate loan programs, 99–100
work-study programs, 98–99
Financial Assistance Available for Graduate Study in Medicine, 107
Ford Foundation, 97
Foreign study programs, 123–138
applying to, 123–125
credit transfers from, 124
language of instruction in, 125
length of education, 124
licensure of graduates, 126–130
number of female enrollments, 4, 5
programs for U.S. medical students, 130–131
Foundations, opportunities for work with, 134–137
Frontiers of Dental Science, 45

G

General Practitioners, 148–152
Genetics, 59
preclinical study program in, 111
Get Ready for College and Go (pamphlet), 99
Giannini, Margaret J., 32–35, 51, 52, 61
Gibby, Mabel K., 65–69, 144
Ginzberg, Eli, 13
Glaser, Helen, 118–119
Green, Gerald A., 75, 85–86
Gynecology
clinical course training, 115
residency requirements, 153

H

Harvard Medical School, 149–150
Hawes, Gene, 23
Health Professions Educational Assistance Act, 105

Health Professions Scholarship Program, 102–104
Hematology, 49–50
Hershey Medical Center, 151–152
High School premedical preparation, 18–21
Histoloty, 111
Honors Program (Northwestern University), 173–176
Horizons Unlimited, 26, 100, 154
How to Pass Medical College Admission Test, 80
Howard University, 76–77

I

Information for United States Students who are Considering Earning a Medical Degree Abroad, 125
Internal medicine
residency requirements, 153
specialization in, 155–156
International Eye Foundation, 135–136
Internship, 139–147
application for, 141
attitudes toward, 147
choice of, 139–140
duration of, 140
duties of, 141–142
for foreign medical graduates, 125–126
mothers, 142–147
part-time programs, 201–202
programs, 200–202
rotating, 139
straight, 139–140
types of, 139–140
vacancies, 140

J

John Hay Whitney Foundation, 103–104
Johnson, Davis G., 10, 74, 224–225
Johnson, Mrs. Lyndon B., 34
Josiah Macy Foundation, 108, 118, 165, 200, 208, 224
postgraduate programs, 192–194
Radcliffe program, 193–194